eXplode: X Fitness Training System

Author: Gino Arcaro

cell: 905-933-7556
email: gino@ginoarcaro.com

Jordan Publications Inc.
Canada

Editor: Janice Augustine
Design: Jessica Ingram
Logistics Manager: Jordan Arcaro
Technical Support: Leeann King

Arcaro, Gino, 1957

ISBN — 978-0-9866191-9-9

Forward

I am addicted to working out.

One of the worst workout addictions in the history of wo/mankind. A seven-day iron-sweat-and-pain addict. I can't take one day off without heavy withdrawal symptoms. Every morsel of food I eat has one purpose – the next workout. Every song on my iPod has one purpose – how it affects my next set. When I go out of town, the first priority is Googling "gyms." Where is the nearest 24-hour gym? Does it have enough free weights? Does it have heavy bags and speed bags? And where can I run? How can I eat enough protein? Packing priorities – workout clothes, iPod and charger, cans of tuna.

My addiction led to starting a business – a 24-hour gym. X Fitness Welland Inc.

I am addicted to being different... thinking so far outside the box that the box disappears. I am deeply committed to not doing things by the book – while writing my own book ... books.

I am addicted to coffee. The intravenous kind. Because it helps fuel my life-long addiction – working out, addicted to the rush.

My greatest fear in life is being bored straight to death and boring others straight to death. It's not an ordinary fear, it's hell. It's connected to an intense aversion to ordinary, routine, mundane, IQ-dropping mind-numbingness. *"Hey, did you hear the one about?"* scares the shit out of me worse than, *"How 'bout that cold?"* The fear of boredom is worse than my other dread – the intense fear of wasting my life, the only life that's been given to me. The fear of spending eternity regretting the trashing of the potential I've been blessed with. The intense fear of replacing destiny with mediocrity. Being asked, *"You work out after midnight?"* is scarier than seeing a ghost but nowhere near as horrifying as THE living-dead question, *"How long 'til you can retire?"*

But my worst addiction, the one I'm most proud of, is wanting to put up ladders for every soul who asks for help. I remain addicted to enjoying the success of anyone willing to take full advantage of opportunities to grow.

I wrote ***eXplode*** to explain my perspective about working out – that it's connected to life performance – how to change what you don't like about yourself. Every human was created for one purpose – to reach full potential. I believe that we have a built-in need to grow. To change. Not simply to re-invent ourselves but to keep adding-on. I believe that we have a natural need to keep building.

eXplode is also a cautionary tale – it's easy to get sidetracked – ignoring our need to change leads to misery. This book is about how to get on track and stay on track. How to exercise free-will. We are blessed with decision-making – the freedom to make the call. Total control in choosing how to respond to everything that happens so that we can make more good things happen.

I know I am not the only addict. I also know that I don't want rehab. I don't need an intervention. I intend to workout hard for the rest of my life. I'll be lifting heavy at 102. Supersets. Dropsets. Megasets.

FORWARD

EXPLODE

"No citizen has a right to be an amateur in the matter of physical training...what a disgrace it is for a man to grow old without ever seeing the beauty and strength of which his body is capable."

- Socrates (469 - 399 BC)

∞

We have been wrongly led to believe that there are only two guarantees in life – death and taxes. Not true. We are guaranteed **opportunity**. Every day, every hour, every minute. Opportunities to improve ourselves and put up ladders for others. Infinite opportunities to do something constructive…as often as we want. And if we don't make it happen, we have no one to blame but ourselves. We can point fingers, complain and make any number of excuses. But trashing opportunity makes us both the perpetrator and the victim of the crime.

Look around at this very minute. With your heart and soul wide open, your mind will follow. You will see what you previously couldn't see…what you refused to see. Life-altering events are patiently waiting for you, sustained by the magic of REPS – opportunity after opportunity to explore your potential, mentally and physically.

There are no limits to opportunities.

I have been blessed beyond all measure to have coached football teams for 40 seasons, thousands of athletes who have joined forces on the field and in the gym to work some magic. Not professional athletes. Students. Not the gifted, talented elite student-athletes… the untalented, ungifted ones looking for a chance – first chance, second-chance, third chance… or more. Grass-roots training – training from scratch. Developing strength physically and mentally in student-athletes who haven't found a place – yet. Young people who have a dream and won't let go of it. I've coached them on the football field and in the weight room, starting in the basement of my house – the original X Fitness where I worked out with each athlete. I never stood by and just watched. I have been eyewitness to miraculous development – young football players who developed into remarkable athletes…beasts. Some went on to the next competitive level on the field but each one without exception went to the next competitive level where it counts most – inside. I'm blessed to have helped them build their inner beast. ***It's truly amazing how a unified team can lift – themselves, each other and any heavy weight that gets in their way.*** I thank God Almighty every day for the opportunity to coach.

I have been blessed beyond all measure to have taught thousands of college law enforcement students in the classroom, to have worked out with those who wanted to separate themselves from the rest, and to have mentored them through an unforgiving hiring process that screens and spits out about 90% of the applicants. I have been eyewitness to miraculous transformation – young students who maximized their opportunities – got into the gym, got hired and developed into currently-serving police officers. I'm truly blessed. I thank God Almighty every day for the opportunity to teach.

I have been blessed beyond all measure to be a gym owner. I started X Fitness from scratch – in my basement. X Fitness is more than a gym. X is a symbol of changed lives… my athletes' and mine. X Fitness reminds me that iron is life-altering. It connects the Big Four – physical, intellectual, emotional and spiritual – a connection I explain in my new book ***Soul of a Lifter***. X Fitness has let me be eyewitness to miraculous development...people who've uncovered their hidden potential to reach next levels and became athletes by the X Fitness definition: anyone who works. Anyone who competes against self, against iron, is an athlete. I'm truly blessed to still be an athlete. I thank God Almighty every day for the opportunity to be a part of X Fitness.

∞

I will never lead my football players or student wannabe cops to get busted up. That's my personal mission statement – to protect them. It's my number one motivation for coaching how I coach and what I coach – on the field and in the classroom. And I can prove it. I have tested every minute detail in ***eXplode***, the X Fitness system and all of it – 100% – has worked to achieve my mandate – to not get people busted up. They don't get pushed around, steamrolled, beaten to the ground, punched out or otherwise get the shit beat out of them. My system builds beasts. Tireless, smart, driven souls with the work ethic of a farm animal. Blue-collar work ethic.

I protect them by teaching them how to outwork their competition. Hard work is feared. Especially the kind of back-breaking work needed to finish a job when fatigue is trying to weaken every mind and muscle fiber. Because those who fear work, especially while under pressure, won't win. Can't win. The Laws of Performance Darwinism won't allow it. How one responds to the pressure of fatigue is the difference between winning and losing – the difference between getting crushed and surviving.

It doesn't matter if I'm preparing athletes to compete in a football game or students to compete in a law enforcement occupation, it's all the same. I seek out the strongest opponent possible then make my team strongest. That's my basic philosophy – call out Goliath then meet him head-on with my inner beast. Merciless, relentless warp-speed attack. Waves of pressure that tire him out then knock him out. Until every Goliath cracks. For over a quarter-century, my track record shows I take the path of **MOST RESISTANCE**...on the field, off the field, in the classroom and in the gym.

My greatest coaching fear is that my football team will quit in the fourth quarter. Not only would it be embarrassing, it would be dangerous. Players could get killed, end up paralyzed, hospitalized or traumatized. Laying down in the fourth quarter is inexcusable. There is no justification for perfectly healthy young athletes to give up when things get tough in the fourth quarter. Left unchecked, quitting before the game is over becomes habitual; it leads to chronic losing, which is carried over to real life and manifests itself in a continued display of unwillingness or incapacity to finish a job. Wannabe cops I've taught know that becoming a quitter can lead to death or serious injury on the job. Letting up in any way in a high-risk sport or job is a sure-fire way to invite disaster. I refuse to contribute to this social mess. Every workout I design is intended to be a ***binding contractual agreement to spill your guts for your teammates. Each workout is a personal investment that binds each member to the team.*** That's why all instruction, on or off the field, starts with lifting heavy – as intense as possible – building an iron-will mindset. The objective of my system is to survive high-risk activities.

But the real measure of the success of a training system is the impact it makes. And to use "impact" as evidence, it must be quantified in terms of "winning." Whether we like it or not, we are judged by our winning record. Winning is the only thing people care about. Winning is not a four-letter word. Winning is not evil. Winning has a broad range of definitions that I discuss throughout this book but the most important part of the definition is this – **survival**... not getting the shit beat out of you on the field, on the streets, or by life in general from the toughest opponent known to wo/mankind... self. *eXplode* makes an impact by building armour – mental and physical armour.

I have been blessed beyond all measure to have worked out for 42 years, no steroids, no interruptions – 100% natural, never taken more than one week off. Four decades of continuous lifting. I'm 54 years old and working out harder, more intense today than ever. My motivation has gone through five stages. First, I needed to end childhood obesity. Second, I needed to excel at high school football. Third, I needed to survive in frontline policing – patrol, SWAT and detective. Fourth, I needed to train my football players and college wannabe cops. Fifth, I needed to not cave in to age. Need it, demand it... the motivational secret that drives all long-term performance and builds the strength to compete on the reality stage, the real-life stage.

But 42 years of working out didn't just happen. Working out is not and never has been a hobby for me, it's a career – one I started in long before becoming an adult. I have been blessed beyond all measure to have had a job in a flour mill throughout my high school days. To have competed in the back-breaking world of manual labour – survival of the fittest – lifting and carrying 140-lb. bags for eight hours every day. Manual labour builds incredible strength and brands you with a blue-collar iron-will tattoo that stays visible for life. The working class teaches you to make it happen through drive, super-commitment and no excuses – just shut up and lift. I thank God Almighty every day for giving me the chance to experience the work behind working out – something I love more than any other part of working out – more than the results and more than talking about it. It helped build an iron-will mindset – the need for the rush. The need for feeling the inner reward of emptying the tank to achieve what I thought couldn't be achieved.

eXplode, the **X** Fitness system has been a work-in-progress for 42 years. Four decades of winning. Four decades of eXploring, eXamining... eXploding. ***A reality show in writing.*** A limitless system consisting of concepts, language and a **Set-Calling©** decision-making model that has been used to design unlimited programs. Limitless ladders to the next levels.

eXplode teaches **functional strength – the practical strength** needed to get a job done – on the streets, on the field, in the factory... any place where you have to make it happen. The X Fitness system strengthens the inseparable connection between mind and body – the one that breaks the barriers that lock up potential.

eXplode is guaranteed to achieve results. Guaranteed to not fail. Guaranteed to succeed...if it's followed precisely.

∞

The secret to life-long workouts is mind-set. Nothing else is more important. Psychology and philosophy are just as important as physiology. Building the mind is just as important as building the body – they're connected. They lift each other. It's impossible to build physical strength (an athletic physique) with a weak mind. Weak mind, weak body.

The leading cause of fitness failure is underestimating the power of the human mind. Not giving the mind enough credit to break past its limits, is limiting. The only reason why fitness goals are not achieved is weak mindset. A soft mind leads to every bad workout habit – poor form, not enough sets, not enough reps, not enough intensity…not enough work. And not enough will power. Left unchecked, a weak mind will stop you from unleashing your full potential… from releasing every ounce of strength and energy you've got locked up deep down in your guts. A weak mind will bury all your gifts and talents. A weak mind doesn't just block your potential… it stops it dead in its track. The mind will quit long before the body does. And it will keep quitting at the earliest sign of discomfort, if you let it. If you tolerate a weak mind, it won't change. It will stay weak. Born weak, stay weak.

How do you change a weak mind? Don't underestimate the mind. Push it. Stretch it. Break limits – smash them… one rep at a time. My job as a coach is to teach hardcore, old-school winning habits that push the weak mind and build mental and physical armour. I start with teaching iron will and beast-of-burden work ethic using the "Big 3" – the primary cornerstones: bench press, squats and wind sprints. I have hardcore beliefs about these Sacred Exercises. I use them religiously, personally and to coach my players. My Sacred Exercises are old-school – basics. I don't debate the merits of military press, bicep curls or anything else I use. There are many secondary Sacred Exercise components that increase balls size while teaching strength, speed, stamina and smarts. But the Big 3 have lifted countless students and athletes to places they had never imagined going.

Here's the controversy – all 3 represent and require extremely hard work. Brutally hard work. **H**eavy **E**xtreme **L**aborious **L**ifting – **HELL**. It's hard to sell any kind of hell. So the hell critics try to challenge the credibility of the Big 3 or invent the Next Big Thing – some replacement for hell, an easier formula for fat loss, bigger muscles and superstar sports performance. Finding the Next Big Thing is a noble effort but the inescapable truth is this: the Big 3 builds armour, builds big balls, and makes an impact. It has transformed horrific losing cultures into winning cultures. My teams' winning record is not stated in terms of championships, of who scored more points in games more often than the competition… our winning record includes a column about life-altering character-building radical mindset transformations that have translated into incredible performances in the gym, on the field, in the classroom and on the streets – functional strength. Practical strength. Strength and conditioning for real-life survival.

PART 1:
THE SYSTEM

What is the X Fitness System? A multi-dimensional strength and conditioning program that includes: lifting in the gym, field running, and motivational learning – fueling the drive. The Psychology, philosophy, and physiology of performance. Mind and body training.

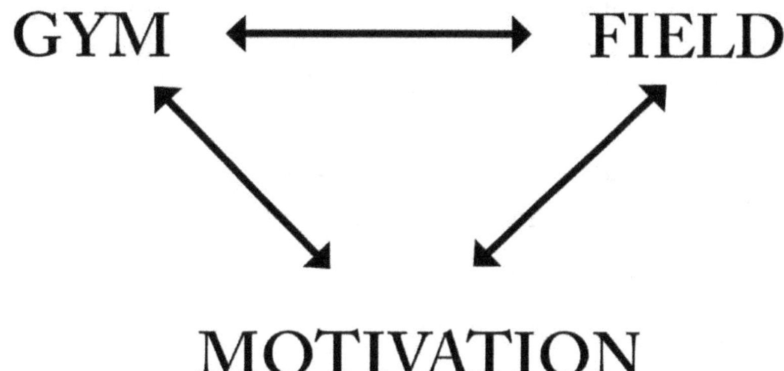

All performance starts at the top, in the mind, and works downward to the body. Positive thinking is not enough. Good intentions alone won't achieve anything. Performance matters. Performance is the universal language that speaks the loudest. Performance is evidence – proof of intention, proof of will, proof of potential, and proof of capability.

I called the system "***eXplode***" because the growth in mental and physical strength of those trained by it has been explosive. I've coached thousands of men and women, using different parts of this system, who experienced explosive transformation in mind and body. It has never been available to the public until now. ***eXplode*** should become your **strength coach** because reaching your full fitness potential is extremely hard to do on your own.

eXplode is unique for 2 reasons:

i. limitless capacity
ii. the ***Set-Calling©*** decision-making model. The science of ***Set-Calling©*** is intended to teach you to:

  » maximize your workouts, and
  » design customized workout programs by ***making the right calls before and during every workout.*** Tailor-made workouts. Workouts that fit your situation. Workouts that fit the moment. ***Set-Calling©*** teaches you how to decide what to lift and when to lift it.

The X Fitness Workout System is the equivalent of a limitless playbook. The system ranges from two extremes – **Power Strength Training to Endurance Strength Training**. The major difference between the two is velocity and workload – workout speed and the length of sustained work – the amount of rest during the workout between sets and the amount of continuous work. **Power Strength Training** features more than one minute rest between sets and single-set format. **Endurance Strength Training** uses supersets and mega-sets with less than 60 seconds rest in between. Power strength training is slower, concentrated on one exercise, and requires short bursts of work with longer rest. Endurance training is faster, spread out, combining multiple exercises to form one set of work, and requiring longer sustained work with shorter rest.

It's impossible to fit every workout I have ever designed and used to build teams or for personal use, in one book. This book explains the basics. It follows a coaching lesson plan, exactly how I have taught it and coached it. Part 1 of the book starts with the final product, examples of two types of program that you can use immediately... two dramatically different workout programs that are part of a larger system. Each specific program combines training concepts that I have developed during my personal workout career and coaching career. Each concept has been tested and evaluated for results, to determine what has worked and what hasn't. I have used my coaching career as a research center.

Part 2 explains the actual X Fitness system, including the philosophy, psychology, and decision-making model that lets you make the right call at the right time.

The first two programs in Part 1 are called:

i. "**1985**" (pronounced nineteen eighty-five)

ii. "**7X7**" (pronounced seven by seven).

I will explain when I use them, why, and for how long. I do everything for a reason. Nothing is done at random. Every workout has a purpose. Every set, every rep, every decision about how much weight to use has a clear purpose. My workouts are not marathons. They're sprints. I accomplish more work in 30 minutes than most people do during 90-minute workouts. My experiments have shown that my athletes dramatically improve on and off the field with short, more intense workouts that dramatically reduce downtime. ***We separate from the rest to separate from the rest.*** Faster workout velocity transforms appearance, strength, stamina, and mindset.

It's important to emphasize that "**1985**" and "**7X7**" are only two examples of concepts within the system, not the whole system. Each represents a point-of-reference to teach and learn the entire system. "1985" and "7X7" give perspective by introducing three elements:

i. language,
ii. concepts, and
iii. decision-making.

And, "1985" and "7X7", which are taught throughout the book in stages, are just two examples that introduce the guts of the system – the 3 Ps:

i. philosophy,
ii. psychology, and
iii. physiology.

My goal in this book is to replicate exactly how I teach and coach — blue-collar work ethic style. No bullshit, just straight from the heart. Like the lessons taught by my hard-working immigrant parents and learned from unforgiving back-breaking manual labour. The single-most powerful lesson of all? **Shut Up And Lift.** Work like a beast, get the job done, no excuses. Nothing transforms mind and body like 8 hours a day of heavy lifting, 5 days a week.

V-Shaped Diagrams

I use several methods to explain a workout. One method is shown in Diagrams 1 and 2 – full or partial V-shaped diagrams with written narratives. I use upright, inverted or half V-shapes to illustrate a graph-like progression of weight, sets or reps. Both diagrams (1 and 2) show half V-shapes, the right side of an upright V that shows an incline in weight. The numbers on the side show a decrease in reps. In other cases, I use only written narratives. Both the V-diagrams and the 100% written narrative will be used to explain the workouts in this book.

The X Fitness system, ***eXplode***, is a direct descendant of the working-class.

Part 1.1:
1985 Concept

Chest

Rounds 1-7 Bench Press – Core workout

Diagram 1

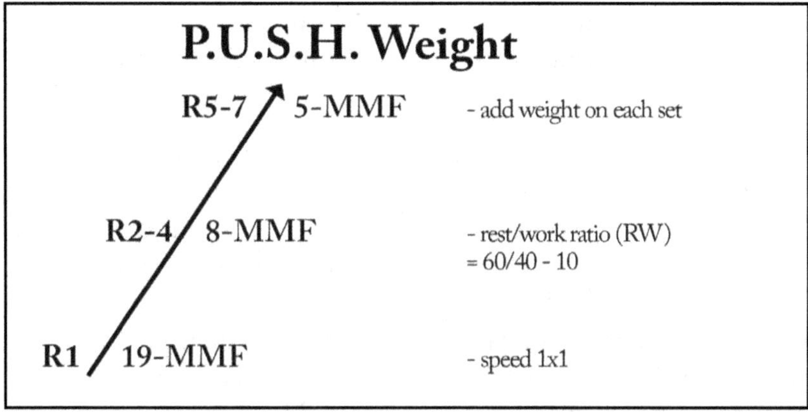

Diagram 2

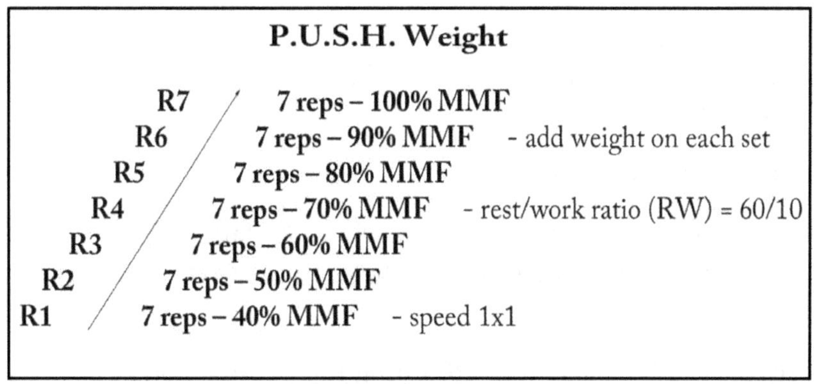

Failure

There's a reason why I chose "1985" and "7X7" to introduce the X Fitness system. They have achieved my coaching goals for my teams and for myself. Secondly, 1985 and "7X7" illustrate the message of my basic work-out philosophy:

- Workouts are a series of <u>failure</u>.
- Workouts are the only job where <u>failure is the goal</u> – not just acceptable, the actual objective.
- The quality of workouts depend on how many times failure is reached during a workout.
- The gym is the only place where <u>total failure is a success</u>.
- Adding up the failures, counts up successes.

- You can't fail all at once. Failure is a step-by-step process. Failure is a work-in-progress.

"Failure" means running out of gas – emptying the tank. Complete failure – 100% failure is lifting a weight until the needle hits "E" and you can't lift any more of that particular weight, in that specific manner, at that moment in time. When the human tank empties, a miracle happens… it re-fills automatically. It takes about 60 seconds to re-fill the tank. The human body is a tribrid – it has three tanks but usually only the first one is used to lift weights and only for about 10 seconds. The other two tanks are generally used for work that takes longer than 10 seconds.

Failure is the secret to fitness success, to strength and conditioning success, to building your intended physique. Failure builds muscle. Failure melts fat. Failure builds stamina. Failure builds iron-will mindset. Failure brings results. Failure makes major changes. Failure transforms. Failure builds success.

Failure is the most important part of a workout because of the workload and the amount of muscle needed to reach failure – more stress on the body, more results. The body has a miraculous way of responding to stress – it adapts to it by building armour. Layers of armour to fight anticipated stress. More armour means leanness and meanness – less fat, more muscle. Chiseled. But armour has a price – hard work. It is a huge investment of exertion but it yields a super-high return – maximum muscular fiber recruitment. Increased workload puts more muscle fiber into play, the equivalent of recruiting an army. And mobilizing it. More troops to do heavy lifting. More troops, stronger force. More muscle fibers recruited leads to more damage which leads to more fibers being repaired and rebuilt resulting in stronger armour.

Failure is Not Created Equal

There's total 100% failure and there's partial failure. It's not reasonable and not possible to achieve 100% failure on every set. ***How many times failure is reached is the workout scoreboard.*** What counts in a workout is:

i. the number of times failure is reached, or

ii. how close you get to failure when you don't reach 100% failure. Complete failures and partial failures – add them up and you calculate the score of a workout… you can figure out if you won or lost the battle.

The cost of making muscle is exhausting – <u>draining the battery</u>. Total 100% failure is the equivalent of letting the battery drain completely to zero. Not 5% or 10%. Zero. Zero is maximum muscular failure (MMF). When the battery reaches zero, the miracle of re-charging fills the battery right back to 100%. But, when the battery re-charges without reaching zero, it won't learn to re-charge fully. Consequently, when zero is never reached, there's a risk that the battery may not charge to a full 100%.

The quality of a workout is measured by how many times the battery is drained, how far it's drained, how fast the battery is re-charged, what we can do with a fully-charged battery, and what we can or cannot do with a partially charged battery. Failure is part of a chain – test the mind, empty the muscle, re-fuel, rebuild.

There are two ways to count partial failure:

i. percentage of complete failure achieved, e.g., 90%; or

ii. percentage of power left in the tank, e.g., 10%.

Both mean the same thing but expressed differently, i.e., 90% failure = 10% power remaining. Like a battery, it's better to drain the human tank to zero. But, unlike a battery, it takes time to condition the human body to go to failure and you can wear out the body by going excessively to failure. Striking the balance is the objective.

In "1985", 100% failure is reached on every set – 100% MMF – 100% sets. In Diagram 1, 100% failure is reached 7 times in 7 sets.

In "7X7", 100% failure is reached only once – the last set. The other 6 sets reach partial failure – close to failure…a percentage ranging from 40%-100% MMF, with partial failure increasing 10% on each set. The "7X7" concept averages 70% MMF, almost three-quarters tank per set, leaving just over one-quarter in the tank.

There's a considerable difference between averaging 100% MMF per set and 70% MMF per set. As this book will teach, a decision has to be made about which one to use – complete failure on every set or partial failure leading up to one set of complete failure. **The right call has to be made to fit the situation.**

"1985" is a grueling, intense ***high-impact*** workout that inflicts a lot of stress on the body. Working out tears down the body causing damage. Recovery repairs and rebuilds. Growth happens during recovery. High-impact means the highest amount of allowable stress and damage. Low-impact means minimal stress and damage.

"7X7" is tough but inflicts 30% less stress. Personally, my decision-making is governed by growth and need. I use the 100% failure per set strategy until growth stops and I need to change. I define growth as lean muscle and strength – the relationship between body-fat and what I can lift. I define need as "need for recovery." I determine this by degree of soreness and post-workout fatigue and how it affects performance. I don't take extended time off. Instead, when I have broken down my body and mind to a point where I need recovery time, I change my workouts to partial failure.

I use the same approach to coaching athletes – fully emptied tanks mixed with partial empty tanks. And with novices, I use a gradual progression from partial failure workouts to full failure – a gradual rise in the partial failure percentage starting at extremely low with minimal increase on percentage failure. A steep incline for novice lifters is a big mistake. Novice lifters cannot work to complete failure right off the bat without learning how to recover from low-impact, low-MMF percentage workouts. That's been my biggest challenge as a strength coach – <u>striking the balance</u> between high-impact and low-impact workouts, for myself and for my athletes.

Striking the balance means walking the fine line between excessive and minimal physical challenge as well as mental challenge – the line between boredom and anxiety.[1] Too little or too much of either boredom or anxiety has the same side-effect – too little growth. Striking the balance is the secret to strength training and strength coaching success. When I've nailed it, explosive growth has happened – teams have transformed into winners, individuals transformed to lifelong workout athletes. When I've blown it, no growth – people quit. The right combination of

1 Tribute to a masterpiece, *Flow: The Psychology of Optimal Experience*, by Dr. Mihaly Csikszentmihalyi (1990). New York: Harper & Row. 'Flow' is winning the struggle between anxiety and boredom which determines the level of performance. Flow is an amazing book. It has been one of the strongest influences that has shaped my coaching and teaching philosophy. I have used Flow in my Master's thesis and partial PhD dissertation, and in every teaching/coaching approach I've used on the field and in college law enforcement classrooms.

complete-failure workouts mixed with partial-failure workouts has been my key to working out uninterrupted for 42 years and the secret to my athletes' strength training success.

Striking the balance is my ultimate objective but it's not easy because striking the balance is personal. It's different for each human. There are too many variables and countless challenges that affect how much we can or can't do in a specific moment in time. But the biggest striking-the-balance problem is underestimating our potential. We can't see our fuel gauge. We rely on our mind and body, in that order, to tell us what's left in the tank. Because of that sequence, we get mixed messages. The mind quits way before the body does – tells us we're on empty when we're not. False fuel reading. Weak mindset – a tendency to underestimate the body's strength capacity and energy source. Left unchecked, the mind becomes a compulsive liar, telling us we've reached failure when we actually haven't. **Underestimating leads to underachievement.**

The accurate test of failure is the body – when the body fails. Real failure means the body cannot lift weight any more at that moment in time – complete 100% MMF. The problem is the body is a follower – a conformist…the body gets influenced too easily and too strongly by the mind. The solution is to strengthen the mind to its potential, stopping the mind from quitting too soon.

The human mind is not born strong. It's born weak. Unless sustained, constructive action is taken, it stays weak. And so the battle rages on – what's the truth, what's a lie. It's one thing to be lied to by others but when the inner voice can't be trusted, we have a problem, a challenge that must be overcome or…we stay weak. **Born weak, stay weak**… that's what I try to prevent in my athletes and myself. My mission is to stop us from staying weak.

There are different paths to failure. Some are more intense than others. Some failure needs more reps than others, some need less. How failure is reached determines how success is reached. "How many reps does it take to reach failure?" The answer lies in which concept I decide to use during the workout. The concepts, "1985" and "7X7", work together to teach the all-important progression that leads to emptying the tank. ***Working out is a series of failures*** – lifting weight until the muscle fails because it runs out of gas. The gym is the only place where failure is a positive. Failure is the pre-requisite to success. But the body needs to be trained incrementally to reach failure. Step-by-step failure conditioning. "1985" and "7X7" form one example of the road to failure.

Dictionary

The X Fitness system has a unique language. The following is an introduction – the basic dictionary. The "1985" and "7X7" concepts are used as points-of-reference to define the language:

- **Core workout**: Main part of the workout.
- **1985**: Concept that leads to 100% failure on every set.
- **7x7**: Concept that goes 100% failure only on one set – the last.
- **Superset**: Two consecutive exercises, zero rest.
- **Mega-set:** Three or more exercises, zero rest.
- **Round:** Group of sets – single-set, superset, or mega-set.
- **Rep speed:** The velocity of lifting and lowering a weight.
- **Rest-work ratio:** A two digit number that shows the relationship between rest and work (in seconds).
- **P.U.S.H.** – **P**erformance **U**nder **S**tress **H**eavyweight. A concept to intensify a workout.

Core Workout: Every workout has a core, referring to the main part of the workout. Diagram 1 represents an example of a CORE workout – the main part of a chest workout that uses the "1985" concept. The core is the primary sets of the bodypart being worked – the center… the foundation. I call the rest of the bodypart exercises the secondary.

The core can be either:

- the entire workout;
- the entire workout for the chest part of the workout with other bodyparts added;
- the main part of the chest workout with other chest exercises added and no other bodyparts;
- the main part of the chest workout with more chest exercises and more bodyparts added.

Examples related to each above:

- 7 sets bench press (core) = entire workout;
- 7 sets bench press (core) + 7 sets shoulders (secondary) = entire workout;
- 7 sets bench press (core) + 3 sets incline + 3 sets decline (secondary) = entire workout;
- 7 sets bench press (core) + 3 sets incline + 7 sets shoulders (secondary) = entire workout;

In these examples, the 7 sets of bench press is the **CORE**, representing the guts of the workout. Whether the core stands alone as the workout for that bodypart or has secondary sets added to it, is a decision based on the past – previous workouts dictate the present. Every workout is connected. Not one workout happens in isolation, separate from past workouts. How I design today's workout depends on what I did yesterday and the days before that. My workouts fit together like a puzzle. They form a string of workouts, like plays called in a football game where each play connects to the next to form a game and games connect to each other to form a season. One set leads to the next. One workout leads to the next. Everything is connected.

"1985": a training concept where 100% full failure is reached on every set, using progressively heavier weight involving a 3-stage **Minimum to Maximum Muscular Failure** **(min-MMF)** rep-range:

- 19 reps min-MMF,
- 8 reps min-MMF,
- 5 reps min-MMF.

19-8-5 min-MMF rep range. All three are minimum, not fixed rep targets. The minimum is a line that must be crossed. The actual finish line is made by your mind, by passing the minimum line and going deeper and deeper. The exercise of free will – you decide how far you can stretch yourself past the minimum.

The goals of "1985" are to:

- Build the blue-collar mindset, a.k.a. the iron-will mindset, the tireless work ethic that breaks barriers to get the job done without excuses. It's the single-most important factor in workout performance.
- Build a base – build or restore muscle memory. Build a neural pathway from scratch or re-inforce a previously built neural pathway that makes a movement second-nature. Build the basics or get back to the basics.
- Train three energy systems. The human body is equipped with the miracle of three energy systems that empty and fill on demand. I group the three systems into two fuel tanks:
    - » 10 seconds and under, or
    - » over 10 seconds.
- Ignite the A-bomb, T-blast, and GH-blast. Unleash the miracle of natural hormones inside our bodies – adrenaline, testosterone, growth hormone. This applies to both women and men. It's the key to peak performance at any age. And it's the anti-aging secret.
- Break limits. Scripted workouts are limiting. Scripted workouts are rigid programs with a fixed finish line – a fixed number of reps that tell you exactly when to stop, when to put down the bar. Scripted workouts don't allow changes to meet changing demands. The problem with scripted workouts is they don't take into account extra strength that may be available to do more reps. Scripted workouts often leave fuel in the tank instead of emptying it. The key to breaking limits is emptying the tank while understanding that the miracle of recovery re-builds, re-fuels, and enlarges the tank. The alternative to scripted workouts is strategize and improvise – make the call to adjust to the situation.

This Core bench press workout has 58 minimum reps over 7 minimum rounds. The objective is to do more reps and more sets if the tank is not emptied. If strength and energy levels are high enough, go past the minimum.

"7X7": a training concept where 100% full failure is reached only once, on the seventh and last set, and partial failure is reached on the six sets leading to the MMF finale. "7X7" uses the same weight and same reps (7) throughout the 7-set sequence. The goal of "7X7" is to train yourself to reach MMF on every set. "7X7" is a strategy that progressively leads up to emptying the tank. It conditions the body to incrementally feel the draining of the battery.

Superset: A superset is two consecutive exercises performed with zero rest (same bodypart or different bodyparts).

Mega-set: A mega-set is three or more consecutive exercises (same bodypart or different bodypart) done with zero rest.

Round: example – R1 -7 (round one –seven): 'R' in diagrams 1 & 2 means "round one to seven." A round is a group of sets, a.k.a set sequence. It can be comprised of only one single-set or multiple sets (supersets or mega-sets). In this example, 7 rounds is the minimum. In diagram 1, each round has only one set of bench press. Diagram 1 features seven rounds with one set in each round.

Rep speed: two digit number, example – 1x1, pronounced one-by-one. Every rep has two-parts: positive (lifting stage) and negative (lowering stage). The first digit refers to the number of seconds for the positive/lift stage of the rep. The second digit refers to the number of seconds needed to lower it. I assign a speed according to what I'm trying to accomplish, for example 2x2, 1x2. Total rep time is calculated by simply adding the two numbers, in other words, total rep time for 1x2 is 3 seconds to do one rep.

Rest-work ratio (RW ratio): a two digit number, example – 60/20. The first digit refers to the rest between sets. The second digit refers to the duration of the set – the total time spent actually working during a single-set, superset, or megaset. The time spent working during a set is an estimate. I don't stare at the clock. I go by instinctive knowledge of time. And, the work-time varies depending on the concept I'm using and what I'm trying to accomplish. For instance, using the "1985" concept, the work-time will vary in accordance with the high reps, mid-reps, or low reps. The speed of each rep depends on the assigned number, ranging from about 40 seconds (19 reps) to 16 seconds (8 reps) to 10 seconds (5 reps). Consequently, the assigned RW ratio varies from 60/40 to 60/16 to 60/10. Because "1985" works to MMF, the work time will increase when more than the minimum reps are lifted.

I decide on the amount of rest (the first digit) between sets according to the purpose of the specific workout. The above example has 60 seconds rest. I lower the number of seconds when my workout goals change. Usually, I use the same rest-between-set time for the entire workout. In some cases, I make the decision to speed up the workout and reduce the rest time separating sets when I'm on fire.

Power Strength Training and Endurance Strength Training have different rest-work ratios. Power strength training has a higher first digit and lower second digit, e.g., 120/5. Endurance strength training has a more balanced ratio, usually with a lower first digit and higher second digit, e.g., 30/60.

P.U.S.H: **P***erformance* **U***nder* **S***tressful* **H***eavyweight*. P.U.S.H is a training concept that adds intensity to a workout by:

- set workload – lengthening the work time of a set. Increasing the amount of continuous work to a set by adding reps or adding workload through continuous work (superset or mega-set); or
- set frequency – reducing rest between sets, or

- set weight – adding weight to the bar, or
- all of the above.

P.U.S.H adds quantity and quality of work by speeding up the workout pace and adding volume of sustained work. This creates a different kind of heavyweight that I call "stressful heavyweight." P.U.S.H tests physical strength by making the weight feel heavier than it is because of fatigue, a safe way to add weight without adding plates. And P.U.S.H tests mental strength by forcing the mind to expect the unexpected. **P.U.S.H. pushes limits**. P.U.S.H. trains body and mind to stay strong longer, to maintain work ethic when the stress of fatigue sets in, to not give into the discomfort of prolonged work, to resist the temptation to cave into the pressure of more resistance, and to NOT QUIT before you have unleashed all your hidden reps. In other words, P.U.S.H. helps significantly in strengthening the mind to not quit.

Psychology of Fatigue

Understanding the psychology of fatigue is crucial to working out because fatigue affects mindset. Mindset is the key to reaching work-out potential and workout longevity. Working out starts at the top – in the mind – mindset. The mind will try to quit at the earliest onset of fatigue, well before all your potential reps are unleashed. Fatigue has to be controlled and managed in order to conquer it before fatigue conquers you.

Fatigue adds weight to the bar without actually adding plates. Fatigue makes the weight feel heavier than it actually is, turning ordinary weight into crushing weight. It's impossible to get stronger and leaner without managing fatigue because ***fatigue is an anabolic agent of weakness.***

The quality of a workout depends on the degree of challenge. The greatest workout challenge is overcoming weakness. Weakness is brought on by real or imagined fatigue. The objective of working out is to manufacture the most stress that fits your situation, then handle it, and overcome it. Stress is manufactured by work – heavy lifting. Hard work brings on fatigue, physically and mentally. If a workout does not challenge you with fatigue, it's not a workout.

The challenge of conquering the loss of physical strength and energy during a workout is the most important element of any workout. To qualify as a challenging workout, the workout has to compete with weakness – bring you face-to-face with weakness and beat it. Push past it. Weakness will test you in every workout if you're training hard enough. If you're not tested by potential weakness, if there is no battle with fatigue, the workout will not achieve the results you want.

Physical fatigue is a tough opponent… a test of what you've got and don't have. But the bigger test is beating the tired mind, the inner voice that uses fatigue to try to convince you to take it easy, relax, or flat out quit way before the tank is empty. The tired mind has one desire – comfort. It will use everything in its power to break your will. Left unchecked, the weak mind will weaken the body. You can measure the challenge and toughness of a workout if your free will gets exercised… if you have to make a decision between two choices – manage fatigue or mismanage it. If there aren't two choices, if you never have to face a test of quitting because of fatigue or weakness, then the workout is not tough enough, not challenging enough, and will not unlock your concealed reps… your full potential.

Fatigue management breaks barriers; fatigue mismanagement breaks your will. Beating fatigue pushes you to higher performance levels. Fatigue mismanagement inhibits progress and growth, promotes weakness and is one of the leading causes of quitting. The secret is to face it – use fatigue as a training partner. Stare at it, don't blink…never run from fatigue. Fight through it. The key is **REPS** – **R**epeated **E**xposure to **P**ressure and **S**tress… train and condition yourself to feel it and beat it.

Psychology of Heavyweight

Heavyweight is not created equal. Neither is **lightweight**. Most athletes I've coached make the mistake of using abstract definitions: ***"That's too heavy. That's too light."*** I've re-defined heavyweight and lightweight with concrete meaning to fit my system.

Lightweight means weight capable of being lifted for over 8 reps, with the last 5 reps leading to MMF.

Middleweight means weight capable of being lifted between 5-8 rep max, with the last 5 reps leading to MMF

Heavyweight means:

- weight capable of being lifted for only 5 reps to MMF (5RM, five reps max). If you can't do more than 5 reps, the weight is heavy; and
- the last 5 reps of lightweight or middleweight that lead to MMF. Any 5 reps that lead to failure is heavyweight . That's the key to the definition of heavyweight. Any 5 reps that lead to failure at the front or back of the set is heavyweight.

Super-heavyweight means one rep max (1RM).

Super-lightweight means any weight that does not lead to failure.

The key point is 5RM-MMF is heavyweight regardless of where you lift it – beginning or end of the set. Five reps max that lead to failure constitutes heavyweight whether it's heavy at the start of a set because of the weight of the plates or if it's heavy at the end of a set because of fatigue. This means:

- Any set that leads to MMF includes heavyweight (e.g., 19 reps that leads to failure include 5 RM at the end, constituting heavyweight).
- A set can start as lightweight or middleweight but can end up as heavyweight because of fatigue, ***if the set leads to failure***. Lightweight and middleweight are starting points. They never finish as lightweight or middleweight ***if failure results.***
- If failure does not happen, the weight is not heavyweight, it's super-lightweight. In other words, if failure happens, there's heavyweight involved. No failure, no heavyweight.

Lightweight and middleweight can change to heavyweight by adding one of two types of stress:

i. higher reps

ii. less rest.

Stressful heavyweight means heavyweight made heavier by doing one of the following:

- reducing rest between rounds to 60 seconds or less; or
- adding supersets or mega-sets; or
- adding plates; or
- all of the above or any two of the above.

Psychology of the "Minimum – Maximum Rule"

The key to continuous natural strength improvement for experienced lifters is creating minimum goals for every workout and then exceeding them. Except for rookies, the biggest mistake lifters make is continuously setting a concrete limit of sets and reps. Creating a rigid, concrete scripted workout does not guarantee physical and mental growth. The secret is setting a minimum, a threshold that must be crossed to determine how far you exceed it to the maximum. It's the equivalent of having two finish lines – a minimum one that must be reached and another one farther past it to test what you're really made of. In other words, the keys to building natural strength are:

- Meet the minimum. Every set, every workout, meeting the minimum is a mandatory starting point.
- Exceed the minimum. Go past the minimum. Break limits.
- The extent that you exceed the minimum determines your strength gains. How far you pass the minimum determines how far you go in the gym. The extent constitutes the maximum. In other words, the maximum should never be predictable. Only the minimum is predictable.

There is a way to keep score to measure if you're winning or losing in the gym. The ***eXplode*** system has a decision-making model that governs how to set the minimum. Combined this with a formula that measures the extent that you surpass the minimum (simply calculate the percentage of additional reps, e.g., 25% more, 50% more, 100% more) and that is your grade...your report card per set. Then add it up for the entire workout to get a score of how far you exceeded the minimum.

Additionally, I calculate total workload of a workout. Single-rep max and the number of reps at 225 lbs. are examples of performance indicators but they are superficial measurements. This means they only measure the surface performance...one moment in time during the workout. To measure deeper, you have to quantify the exact workload performed during the entire workout. Performance indicators measure a narrow performance within the context of the workout but not the entire context. The total workload is the context – the complete measurement – that's what matters. That is the real game. How to calculate total workload will be explained in Part 2.

The strength training game is about who wins the quantifiable total workload during a concrete training period. But ultimate success in strength training is simply staying in the game. As long as you're in the game, you are not a failure...unless you never reach failure.

Psychology of "Tired Work"

The rest between sets determines the quality of work, meaning performance that is stressed under fatigue or not. There's a big difference between rested work and tired work. Performance at the start of a game, or start of a shift, or start of a workout is expected to be impressive because the tank is full – the battery is charged. During a football game, the first quarter performance is expected to be high-level – both teams are at their strongest. During the first quarter of a police patrol shift, officers are expected to work hard because fatigue has not set in. In the gym, we are supposed to be strong during the first quarter of a workout. And, the first half is supposed to be easier than the second half. The second half is a test of mental and physical strength. But the **4th quarter** goes deeper. The **4th quarter** separates winners from losers. The **4th quarter** is the ultimate test of will-power. It shows what you're made of. Positive thinking is not enough. The **4th quarter** forces you to prove who you are, forces you to present the evidence of what you've got. He/she who asserts must prove.

My objective for my teams and myself is simple – strength when tired and strength while rested must be at least equal. This means there can't be a drop off in 4th quarter strength. Staying strong in the 4th quarter is not an option. It's not a choice. It's not an alternative. Staying strong in the 4th quarter is a necessity. And, 4th quarter performance should reach higher. Raising the bar in the 4th quarter is the true measure of a winner – a champion.

Caving in in the 4th quarter is a danger, whether on the field or on the front-lines or in the gym. The risk of getting badly hurt increase when the mind and body weaken. Weak-will will risk your safety. Weak-will will get you hurt. Weak-will will make you lose. When the competition stays strong in the 4th quarter and you weaken, then the dreaded <u>mismatch</u> happens. Mismatches get ugly. The mismatched don't just lose, they get hurt. In any job or sport, equally-matched opponents may seem like a fair fight at the start of the first quarter. Equal-strength in the 1st quarter does not guarantee equal strength in the 4th quarter. The real opponent is fatigue. The tired mind is the true enemy. Unbalanced fatigue tilts the playing field. When one side stays strong longer, the effects of the mismatch become greater. Mismatches lead to misery. To survive, mismatches must be prevented. The moment that the tired mind starts sending signals of doubt and fear, we're in trouble. Decision time – we have to make a tough call…give up or give all.

There are two types of weakness that affect any performance:

i. full-strength weakness: the soft parts we start the first quarter with – the weaknesses we haven't knocked out yet, and

ii. fatigue-weakness: softness that develops when our minds and body get tired.

Fighting through "tired work" builds character, mindset, muscle, balls… everything needed to win. A phenomenon happens when we fight through fatigue – we lift performance during tired work to the same level as performance during rested work… or higher.

Psychology of "P.U.S.H."

Currently, I use Endurance Strength Training, featuring low rest range (between zero-60 seconds) and higher sustained workload. During the first two decades of my workout career, I used Power Strength Training, featuring upper rest-ranges between 3-5 minutes because lifting single-rep maximum (1RM) was one of my top priorities. Routinely, I tested strength two ways:

- 1RM - lifting as much weight as possible for one rep, and
- lifting 225 lbs. for as many reps as possible. Bench press, squats, and deadlifts were three exercises that tested 1RM and 225 lbs. reps. Three to five minutes rest just before the testing set worked wonders. Single-rep max served its purpose – power and strength, mentally and physically. In fact, there's no rush that compares to successfully lifting 1RM contests with self. But, a price is paid to lift 1RM naturally for years, without steroids and without performance-enhancing drugs. Two build-ups happen – the build-up of wear, tear, and injuries and the build-up of bulk. For my first two decades, I ignored soreness, hurt, and outright pain – it was all part of the game. And it was worth it. Lifting 1RM makes you feel as strong as a beast of burden, as tough as a brick wall, and indestructible. For football and frontline policing, it was the building blocks of deep-rooted confidence – real self-assurance, a feeling of self-reliance and self-security that can't be matched. Power strength training got the job done.

Endurance Strength Training. After I left policing, I continued 1RM but with less frequency. I still used 1RM to coach my athletes so they could enjoy the benefits of raw strength on the field but my focus started to change from 1RM to 5RM as the new benchmark, along with stressful heavyweight, and continued 225 lbs. testing. I used the third decade of my career to make that transition that eventually changed my training ideology and transformed my physique. High intensity has always been a trademark of my workouts, even during the 1RM part of my career. But, as I phased out 1RM, the intensity reached higher and higher levels, cutting up my bulk without sacrificing 225 lbs. strength. In decade four, I occasionally gave in to temptation and tested myself at 1RM but I dramatically shortened the rest between sets down to 60 seconds, 45, 30, sometimes zero, using abs as the only bodypart rest at the end of a superset or mega-set, making the weight feel heavier and heavier but without the injuries.

Additionally, my lifting career has corresponded with my football coaching career. During my 1RM phase of my workout career, I was a ground & pound coach on both offense and defense. Run the ball and stack the line. Single-rep max was compatible to my on-field ideology. As I transitioned away from 1RM to a more intense 5RM & 225-oriented philosophy, I made the change to a warp-speed no-huddle featuring high-octane passing on offense and heavy blitzing on defense. Strength was still the key but the emphasis changed to leaner, faster, meaner, and... tireless. Stamina and strength. **Endurance.** It worked. Outworking your opponent with continuous warp-speed relentlessness, instead of short bursts of energy, tilts any playing field – sports or real-life. **Endurance is the secret to winning in sport and real-life.** Outlasting the competition is the way to compensate when you're mismatched. **Endurance training does not replace strength training...it adds to it, building onto strength training. Endurance strength training** revolutionized my teams' performance, my own performance, and our collective appearance. Slow strength training has a purpose. So does faster strength training. The X Fitness system is a limitless system that includes both.

Zero to sixty changes fueling time tank size. Sixty seconds is now my magic number for rest between sets. Sixty seconds is my upper limit. It's the most amount of rest I ever take because 60 seconds is all it takes for the miraculous human tank to be filled. Sixty seconds charges the battery. Anything more than 60 seconds is counter-productive and a waste of time for what I'm trying to accomplish for my athletes and myself. But, I rarely use the full 60 seconds. The reason is that I have trained myself and my athletes to stay stronger longer with 45 seconds rest and less. I don't have the medical evidence to support this next claim but I have anecdotal evidence based on recorded performance – ***I believe working out faster trains and conditions the body to fill up the tank faster and, expands the tank size.*** The battery-charger gets faster and becomes more powerful, needing less than 60 seconds to reach 100% full while also increasing battery life. To emphasize this point, here's my evidence – ***similar performances with 60 seconds rest and under 60 seconds rest.*** I have been recording the performances of countless athletes I've coached since I started strength coaching in "1985" and my own performances since I started working out in 1969. What I found was that repeated high-intensity training with 45 seconds rest or less resulted in similar test scores when 60 seconds rest was taken. The key is repeated intense training – repeatedly reducing the rest time to intervals between 45 and 60 has not diminished strength but actually maintained it. Tests I routinely conduct have shown that we can lift the same amount of weight with less rest time if we get conditioned to it. The benefit of faster, higher intensity is more fat burned, more muscle, tougher mind – more work, more reps, less time equals more fat loss physically and mentally. Leaner and meaner.

Under 60 seconds rest between sets is a test of ***fatigue management***, where I teach how to ***perform under fatigue***, lift without a full tank while training the body to fill the tank in less than 60 seconds, and most importantly, how to conquer the weak mind…how to get the mind in shape, how to condition and train the mind to break its habit of pessimism, how to transform the mind from a negative source to a positive one

This book series explains the old and new – 1RM and no 1RM but I will work in reverse, from the present to the past. The workouts will start with the faster, more intense P.U.S.H concept to the slower, power-based 1RM series.

P.U.S.H. Weight, P.U.S.H. Reps. The P.U.S.H. concept can be applied with or without adding weight. There are two ways to **P.U.S.H.:**

i. add weight and rest 60 seconds or less

ii. use the same weight, reduce rest between zero and 60 seconds using supersets and mega-sets, and increased reps.

P.U.S.H. Weight means **"add weight + reduce rest under 60 seconds."** The goal of P.U.S.H. Weight is to make the weight heavier by the combined effect of added plates and reduced rest. P.U.S.H. Weight also means lowering the minimum rep range (e.g., from 19 to 8 to 5).

P.U.S.H. Reps means **"lift the same weight with less rest."** Instead of adding plates, add the stress of fatigue. A phenomena happens. The number of reps grows. When you lift the same weight over and over, two miracles happen:

i. muscle memory – the miracle of neural pathways builds second-nature, automatic pilot, machine-like lifting, and,

ii. conditioning manages fatigue. Fatigue decreases instead of increases. You stay stronger longer.

This rep-building phenomenon has been the secret to dramatically increasing all-important reps at 225 lbs., the litmus test for football players to prove their physical and mental strength in order to move to the next level. Scholarships and pro contracts are at stake. Adding reps to 225 lbs. testing is a major part of the X Fitness system. It's the key to reach higher professionally and personally but it also transforms body and mind. Adding reps at 225 builds lean muscle – burns fat... chisels and shreds.

What if you don't have the body-weight to rep 225 lbs.? The X Fitness system includes an alternative weight for undersized lifters of both genders. In other words, the system can achieve the incredible benefits of high-rep heavyweight lifting by using less than 225 lbs., based on a formula that will be explained later in the book.

Part 1.2:
Reading Diagram 1 – 1985 Concept

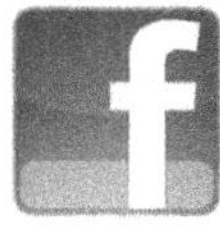

X-Fitness Welland

The human body will take immediate action and will look the way you want it to look if you lift something heavy enough times and fuel it with a high-octane blend.

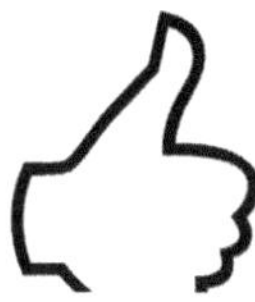

Craig Shiloh Carsty, Ahmed Muktar and 6 others like this.

1985 Concept — Chest

Rounds 1-7 Bench Press – Core workout

DIAGRAM 1 (SAME AS PREVIOUS DIAGRAM 1)

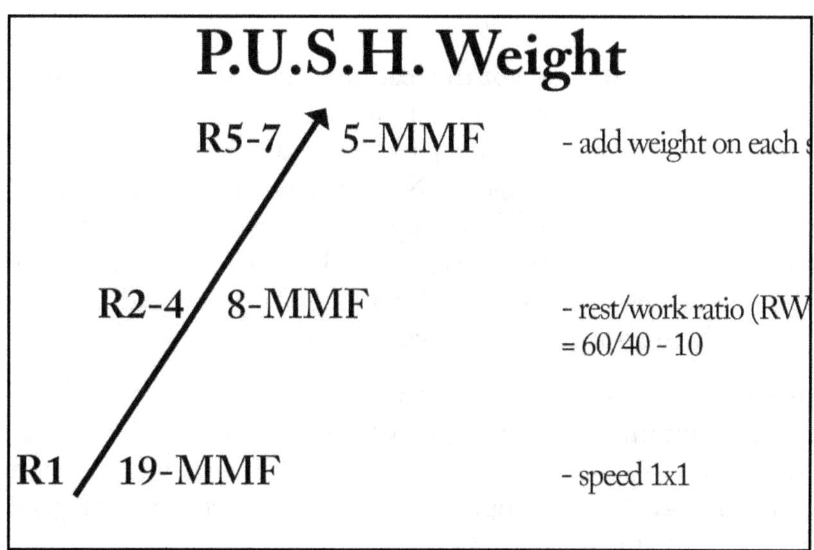

Instructions:

This diagram illustrates the core of a chest workout – 7 sets of bench press using the "1985" concept, single-set format. The core workout can stand alone or it can be built on – connected to other chest exercises or other bodypart exercises.

7 single-set rounds. Each round consists of a bench press set. No supersets, no mega-sets in this diagram. Later in the book, the intensity of this chest workout will be increased by adding supersets or mega-sets.

The arrow rising at a 45-degree incline shows how the P.U.S.H. Weight concept will add weight to each set. One of the objectives is to add weight for each set and progressively reduce reps.

Round 1 – The first set is a minimum of 19 bench press reps lifted to 100% failure. Don't put the bar down at 19 reps unless you've reached complete failure. If you have not reached 100% failure at 19, do more reps. The purpose of 19 reps is:

- blood flow – preliminary pump. This not a warm-up set. I don't use the word "warm-up" because warm-up implies a comfortable rep that does not reach failure. 19 reps will flood the chest with blood, starting the pump process.
- **Neural pathway** – whether you're a novice lifter or an expert lifter, high reps will forge neural pathways (referring to connections between the brain and nervous system) resulting in muscle memory...second-nature movement. Automatic pilot. Lifting without thinking. Neural pathways are the key to lifting the heaviest weight of all – **fear**. Fear and anxiety are the strongest performance blockers – specifically, fear that the bar will crash down and crush you. Holding a heavy weight over your chest is intimidating unless it's routine and deeply familiar. Uncertainty causes performance-paralyzing fear. Familiarity removes fear by converting uncertainty to certainty. The only way to make anything routine and familiar is **REPS** – **R**epeated **E**xposure to **P**ressure and **S**tress. Face up to the pressure and stress of holding a heavy bar over your chest by repeatedly lifting it up and down. Do it over and over, countless times. High reps is crucial to forming muscle memory so that the act of bench pressing, or any other type of lift, becomes second-nature. A minimum of 19 reps accumulates over time to form solid neural pathways to make you fearless of the bar.
- **Work ethic** – weak work ethic is one of the leading causes of lifting failure. Laziness is real, there's no other way to put it. It is the biggest factor that affects workout success. Laziness is part of human nature's constant search for pleasure, and pain avoidance, all of which leads to work-aversion... a repugnance for exertion. No one is born with a strong work ethic. It has to be developed – taught and learned. The only way to develop a strong work ethic is to face repeated challenges of demanding workload...sustained work – working harder. longer. Sets of minimum 19 reps teaches the demands of working for prolonged time periods. High reps test the mind and body to go where they have not been.
- **Feeling 20 reps** – bench pressing 225 lbs. for reps is the litmus test for football testing of upper body strength. A minimum of 19 reps forces the lifter to lift 20 or more reps. Twenty reps is the threshold that separates ordinary lifters from extraordinary lifters. Every set that a lifter reaches 20 reps, ***at any weight***, is an opportunity to experience what it feels like, mentally and physically to lift a weight at least 20 times.
- Manufacture fatigue to make the last 5 reps heavyweight. The first 14 reps are intended cause fatigue for two reasons:

  i. to learn how to work through fatigue, and

  ii. to make the last 5 reps feel heavy. The objective is to convert the 19 rep minimum into a 5RM set. Change the focus, change the outcome. I teach that a19-rep set is actually a stressful 5RM set. It's not a light set, not a "warm-up" set, it's a heavy set... a unique way to lift a stressful 5RM heavyweight by doing 14 reps, getting tired, and finishing with a fatigued 5RM.

- Weight selection – how much weight do you lift for round 1? The answer is calculated by studying yourself, by acknowledging current strength and past strength. Research is the key. Experiment. **Study yourself.** Learn your strength. Understand it. **Quantify your strength.** Record your workout performances. Write notes ***after*** the workout, not during – the reason is focus. Writing during a workout breaks focus and reduces intensity. Knowing you have to write notes afterward dramatically increases focus and memory recall. Keeping a notebook is your research. It's the only way to make the right calls about weight selection. **It's impossible to know how much weight to put on the bar without studying yourself.**

All bench press weight selection has a relationship with bodyweight – a percentage of body-weight is chosen for every set. Veteran athletes I coach are expected to know what weight to select for each minimum standard – 19,8,5. Begin with a warm-up of a minimum of 19 pushups, hands positioned directly under shoulders - not wider, not narrower. My personal weight selection for the first set is 120 % body-weight (BW). In my case, 225.lbs. That first set weight took me a decade to reach. You don't get there overnight.

If you're a rookie lifter (male or female) and have not studied yourself, use the following first-set formula: 25% body-weight (BW) for min 19 reps. I define a rookie as any lifter in his/her first year of true working out, true lifting. Gym experience is not created equal. I don't count unchallenging, unstructured lifting experience when I interview athletes. ***"I've been working out three years"*** often translates to cumulative rookie experience – a few months at best. A rookie has three characteristics:

i. weak mind

ii. weak body, and

iii. horrible form and technique.

A rookie fears the bar, consciously or sub-consciously, manifesting in a wide range of odd behaviours and statements. My research shows that 25% BW for a rookie's first set lets him/her rep-out past 19 reps to achieve all the goals of a 19-rep minimum set.

Round 2 – In this workout, the rest-work ratio for round 1 is 60/40. This means that 19-reps min. will take about 40 seconds of sustained work, and 60 seconds rest will separate the first and the second set/round. There are variables that affect the 40-second workload, including maximum reps and pace. 40 seconds of work may be longer depending on the pace of the lifting and the number of reps that you go past the minimum. Lifting pace is an inexact science. The velocity that a bar is lowered and lifted is an approximation. It's impossible to count seconds while lifting and lowering heavy weight. I teach fast-speed (1x1) to train explosion used in football and slow-speed (2x2) to recruit more muscle fibers. But I never consciously count seconds, not during my lift or my athletes' lifts. Fast-speed and slow-speed are great teaching instructions. A long set includes both fast-speed and slow speed. The pace is affected by the extent of fatigue – my pace is slightly faster during the first half of a long set, slightly slower in the second-half of the set but always under control. I train my athletes for explosion and control of the bar, which translates to a starting 1x1 pace that gradually changes to 2x2. Consequently, the first set workload time aims for 40 seconds but may increase depending on how far I go past the minimum.

During the 60 second rest, another decision is needed for the second round weight selection. Round 2 calls for a minimum of 8 reps to MMF. Enough weight has to be added to build the 8-rep threshold and cross it, pushing out more reps to failure. The psychology of the "minimum rep threshold" forces the lifter to break past limits. Select enough weight to make the 8-rep min. challenging enough. Then pass it. The last 5 reps have to lead to MMF so the 5RM is reached. The 8-set minimum must include the stressful heavyweight of a 5RM to failure at the end of the set.

This weight selection decision needs personal research, just like in Round 1. Study yourself. As a general rule 10% more weight works. The energy expended by the first set combined with only 60 seconds rest and a 10% additional workload achieves the 8-rep min. challenge. But you have to experiment to find the right percentage of weight to add.

Round 3 – The rest-work ratio for round two is 60-20…about 20 seconds of work followed by 60 seconds rest. Make the call during the 60-sec. rest time. The P.U.S.H. Weight objective calls for adding weight while keeping the same 8-set minimum. A phenomenon happens after 2 rounds – strength builds instead of diminishes. Two rounds accumulate a minimum of 27 reps with 60 seconds rest separating the 27 reps and another 60 seconds following the 27th rep. Both rounds will have included a 5RM stressful heavyweight to failure. All of this leads to strength deficit management, referring to the proper management of strength loss – preventing weakness. This routine manages fatigue. Instead of getting tired, you get stronger. Consequently, for this workout, I use the same 8-rep minimum for round/set 3. You can select heavier weight and still reach and pass the 8-rep minimum. The "study yourself" rule still applies but as a generally speaking, a range of 5-10% increase applies.

Round 4 – The same round 3 narrative applies – word-for-word.

Rounds 5-7 – After 4 rounds, you should be on fire. Your strength levels should be on the rise. The minimum total reps for the first 4 rounds is 43 reps. During those 4 rounds, you will have lifted 5RM stressful heavyweight four times. Don't confuse this with a "warm-up," a fire has been built deep inside, a power that replaces any hint of weakness with strength… ***if you train consistently.*** Continuous training is the key. It's impossible for performance to exceed training. Fight like you train, train like you fight.

After 43 minimum reps in the "1985" progression, you are now prepared for the **4th quarter performance**, where you will break past previous limits. Fourth quarter performance separates ordinary and extraordinary, transforms a winning culture from a losing culture, and makes the step-by-step climb to reaching higher. You can't stay in one place in the gym. You go higher or lower – your choice…depends on fitness, how you exercise free will.

The last 3 rounds sets are 5RMs…tests of pure strength, mentally and physically. These 3 sets will pressure and push your body and mind. The physical and mental pump will be off the charts. The sense of accomplishment will be unrivaled.

The RW (rest/work) ratio changes dramatically in rounds 5-7. The workload generally lasts in the 10-second range. Each round is strictly separated by a maximum of 60 seconds. The objective for rounds 5-7 is simple – do not fail to achieve 5RM but don't make it easy. Weight selection is the key. Once again, study yourself. Experiment. Find the percentages of bodyweight that you can lift for at least 5 reps but the weight must be progressively heavier – heavier than the 8-set minimum in rounds 2-4 and progressively heavier throughout rounds 5-7. All this leads to the 5RM test – what can you lift for 5RM. The 7th set is the magic number. Weight selection for the 7th set is a crucial decision. Too heavy or too light defeats the purpose of the "1985" concept. It's important to again emphasize that five reps is the minimum. Don't stop at five if you can do more. Add weight from the sixth rep and add weight from the last bench press workout. Always try to keep setting personal bests. Even if it's a few pounds, keep striving to break your personal record book.

The 7th set. Every athlete I've coached has reached personal bests on the 7th set. The 7th set has been the key to our team successes. Every limit we've broken on the 7th set has translated to limits broken on the field, on the streets, in real-life because the 7th set is a ***fortest***, a word I've developed to define a ***test that builds new strength.*** The word "fortest" combines ***forte*** (Italian for "a strength") and ***test.***

Decades of X Fitness experimentation and research has shown that the performance and result of the 7th set outmatch any other set – no contest. No other set has come close. The 7th set rule has applied to every lift, not just bench press. I have a list of ***sacred lifts*** that form the guts of the system...the basics. Sacred exercises are divided into primary exercises and secondary exercises that are explained later in the book. Every primary exercise has undergone a fortest, where we build new strength by lifting 5RM or 1RM for personal bests. The 7th set rule has applied to both 5RM and 1RM. As stated earlier, my focus has changed to 5RM but the 7th set rule has worked for both.

Why has the 7th set been the peak of lifting performance.? Why the 7th set, and not the 6th of the 8th? I've concluded the following from my research. A minimum of 53 reps spread over 6 sets, including six stressful heayweights of 5RM, produces the chain of 3 F's needed to max out on the 7th – fire, focus, fearlessness. All three are connected. Fire means more than warmed up, more than pumped up...it means a blazing deep-rooted need to push past a limit, break it, shatter it to pieces. Focus refers to the burning concentration needed to lift heavyweight. Fearlessness means the absence of anxiety, apprehension and all the blockers of potential. It's impossible to lift heavy weight without the confluence of a raging fire, burning concentration, and paralyzing fear of the bar. The 7th set has proven to be the perfect moment for a test of strength. The road leading up to it has proven to be the best for managing both fatigue and strength deficit.

This core workout can be a full workout on its own or the core of an extended workout. I rarely use this as the full workout. I have used it for rookie lifters in the off-season or in-season workouts to ensure peak strength levels. Building on to the core is the product of my decision-making process that I call **Set-Calling©**, a formula that guarantees making the right call at the right time.

Part 1.2.1:
Set-Calling©: A Decision-Making Model

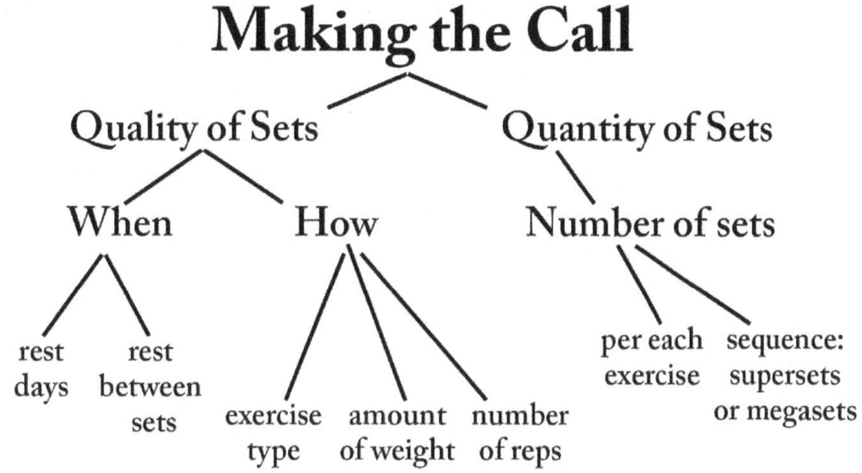

Making the Call

- Quality of Sets
  - When
    - rest days
    - rest between sets
  - How
    - exercise type
    - amount of weight
    - number of reps
- Quantity of Sets
  - Number of sets
    - per each exercise
    - sequence: supersets or megasets

Workouts are a series of decisions, a chain of decisions that form a continuum from workout to workout. Every rep, every set, every workout is connected. No one rep or set or workout happens in complete isolation. Therefore, winging it doesn't work. Decisions need reasoning and logic to make the right call to fit the situation. The **Set-Calling©** model was designed for that purpose.

Understanding the Set-Calling© Model

Scripted workouts are limiting. It's impossible to predict every single moment during a workout, before the workout. That's why it's impossible to script a workout with 100% accuracy for yourself or someone else. It's impossible to predict how you will respond to a 3rd superset, or a 4th mega-set. It's impossible to predict how you will respond to the 7th set. It's impossible to predict how strong or weak you will be after every set. Whether you are coaching a team or coaching yourself, you will not know strength levels during a workout until you get there.

Scripted workouts underestimate strength. Coaching has taught me that humans are poor judges of strength. We have a tendency to underestimate our inner strength, our outer strength, our mental strength, and our metal strength. When a scripted workout instructs fixed reps for a specific set, that's all you will likely do even if you can do more. You will probably follow the instructions and finish the set without emptying the tank. Putting down the bar too early hides reps. Buries them. Concealing reps is a disservice to self – it hides your talent. Unfulfilled reps, unfulfilled potential. Every workout has a full potential…a destiny of its own. The secret is to reach it every time. Unfulfilled reps accumulate, piling up like a heap of trash. Waste.

Calling the right set during a workout is exactly the same as calling the right football play during a game, or making the right decision at a call in policing during an emergency – information has to be instantly processed to evaluate the problem and select the best solution. No time-outs, no time for conference calls, no time to Google the answer. The only way to make tough calls in the heat of the action is **REPS** - **R**apid **E**xtreme **P**roblem **S**olving. Every decision made without the luxury of consultation time, research time, or meeting time is an exercise in REPS. It applies in the gym, on the sidelines, and on the streets.

REPS needs two components:

i. a general plan, and

ii. the capacity to adapt to the unexpected, unpredictable. Expecting the unexpected in not enough. You have to be able to adapt to the unexpected. To do this, you need a system that allows you to change without change – change direction without changing the system… make instant decisions that fit the situation.

A scripted workout rigidly instructs exactly how many sets, how many reps, and what exercises to do. They do have a purpose in guiding rookies, recovering from an intense phase, and in-season training. Otherwise, a script sets limits. Scripted workouts that set an unchallenging finish line defeat the true purpose of working out…to challenge mind, body, soul, and spirit.

Instead of a scripted workout, I use the **strategize & improvise** method that I've named **Set-Calling©**. A concrete decision-making model that leads to making the right calls by general planning and adaptation...a flexible plan that changes to fit the situation. A contextual plan that is customized for a specific moment in time.

Strategize & improvise does not mean unscripted. I never have and never will use an unscripted workout. I design a structured program for every workout, mentally, but without a rigid script. Structured and scripted are two separate concepts. I use the same method that I use in football – a general game plan that builds a framework within which calls are made.

A framework is what the word suggests – a pre-conceived plan that frames the work intended to be performed, leaving room for the pieces inside the frame to change. Flexibility within structure. The frame is the structure, the picture inside it is flexible. **Set-Calling©**, strategizing and improving, and frame-working have been the secret to coaching teams of athletes at the same time – several athletes at the same time without interruption. One of my objectives is eliminating down-time, the needless idle time that destroys the full potential of a workout. The system lets me make rapid-fire calls for the entire team and myself without sacrificing intensity, the speed of the workout, and the crucial flow that sets mind and body on fire. It builds the all-important burning focus that leads to fearlessness...that crucial mindset transformation that separates first-stringers from bench-warmers and a winning culture from losing culture. Fearlessness is not the elusive 100% absence of fear. It's not a tattoo, not a catchy slogan on a T-shirt. **It's managing, channeling, transforming, and unleashing every prior weakness, anxiety, and limiting belief that seek to lock up mind and body – changing us into the force of nature we were intended to be.**

Building sets onto the core workout is a science especially if you're working out while coaching people. I workout alone and with teams of people. I have never coached athletes in the gym from the sidelines. I coach them from the bench...on the bench. This poses my biggest coaching challenge – how to build onto my workout and my team's workout; how to achieve our goals while making call after call for my athletes and myself, all without dropping F-BOMBS – fire, focus, fear, flow, fatigue, framework... the chain of success. Dropping F-bombs means mismanaging one or more F-links. The challenge of strength coaching yourself and/or a team is never breaking the chain of success by dropping an F-bomb.

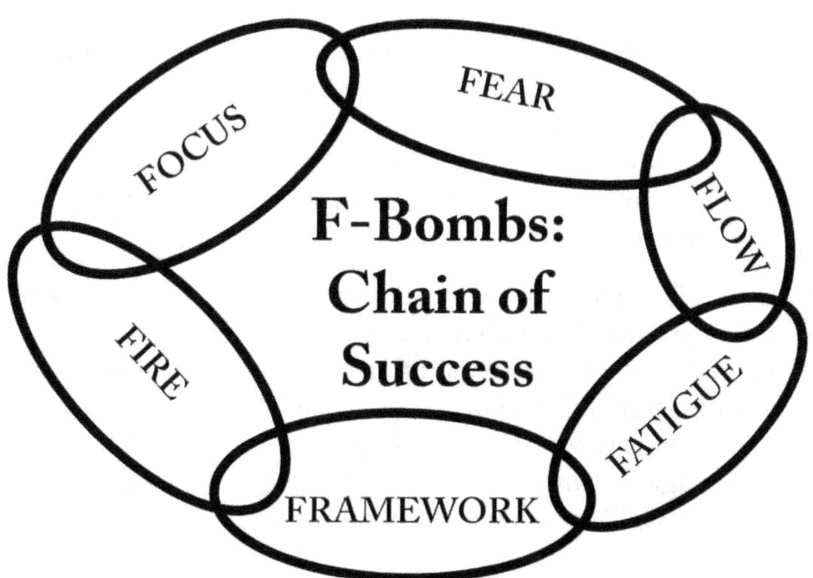

I never workout with a clipboard. That's my number one **Set-Calling©** rule. I never have and never will hold any paper, notebook, clipboard, cell-phone, tablet, white-board, or any other gadget during a workout. Instead, I use the hands-free method to make the calls. It's impossible to build the level of intensity needed to reach the full potential of a workout by carrying around literature during a workout. No notes, no references, no books, no reminders. Everything is stored in my memory. Every call is made without having to read one word… hands-free decision-making. Reason? To prevent distracted workouts.

Like distracted driving, distracted work-outs are dangerous and counter-productive. Distracted workouts kill the drive, wreck the motor, and prevent you from getting where you want to go. Lifting heavy weight is serious business. It's risky and extremely hard. Working out demands 100% focus – a burning concentration, tunnel vision. Two reasons why:

i. what you focus on grows, and,

ii. focus doesn't just happen.

Growth and focus are connected. They're directly proportionate. One promotes the other. A cycle of cause and effect. Focus on anything good or bad and it is guaranteed to grow. When anything grows, so does the focus on it. Broken focus is a leader in the failure business – it's one of the main causes of failure to reach failure and a leading cause of losing in any business…sports, work, personal life, team. Focus is the secret to success in anything we do. What you learn to focus on spreads to your life outside the gym. Focus is transferrable – conditioning yourself to focus intensely during workouts transfers to every other aspect of your life, professionally and personally. Focus builds strength, builds muscle, and tears down fat. Weak focus, weak mind…and weak body.

Any high-risk activity combination demands hands-free decision-making. Distractions break the chain. Distractions drop F-Bombs. I use the hands-free rule to coach football and in the gym, but I learned it originally in policing. At domestics, disturbances, 911 calls, you can't carry a clipboard and read notes while you're trying to make the right call in the blink of an eye.

Calling the right set is the same as calling the right football play and making the right decision at a call in policing – information has to be instantly processed to evaluate the situation and select the best solution. The only way to get better at hands-free decision-making is **REPS** - **R**apid Extreme **P**roblem **S**olving. Every decision made without the luxury of consultation time, research time, or meeting time is an exercise in rapid extreme problem solving. It applies in the gym, on the sidelines, and on the streets.

It's impossible to accurately predict the effects of exertion and hard work with 100% certainty. Extreme exertion is a change agent – it either strengthens or weakens but you cannot make an accurate 100% prediction. I have been asked thousands of time, "***Can you write a workout for me?***" It's impossible to script a meaningful workout without knowing and, more importantly, understanding that person's precise workout history leading to his/her current strength level. Writing workouts without an investigation into the lifter's past is blind coaching. The solution is collaborative coaching – joint **Set-Calling©**. Strength coaching any female or male lifter, I teach them how to make their own calls.

I do the same in football. I designed a warp-speed no-huddle offense where the quarterback and coach share play-calling – the coach starts the play and the quarterback finishes it. This system leads to the quarterback learning to make his own calls from the system. Learn and lead. ***Independent decision-making*** is the secret to high-level performance. I learned in policing that a supervisor cannot and will not hold your hand on every call after you graduate from rookie status. Rookies are taught how to make the tough calls with the expectation that they will make them alone. Same with football. I teach the quarterback how to make calls but eventually he has to do it on his own. Independent decision-making at the right moment is key to optimal growth – intellectually and physically.

The same applies to working out. I coach rookies by making the calls for them until they learn to make their own decisions. Independent **Set-Calling©** starts with weight selection. Rookies become responsible for learning how much weight to put on the bar. REPS make **REPS - Rapid Extreme Problem Solving** makes a **R**eal Expert **P**roblem **S**olvers. Never forget that every work-out is a problem-solving exercise, an investigation where you're trying to solve the mystery of building peak strength, peak physique, and peak performance.

The next section of this book explains how I apply **Set-Calling©** to build on to the core work-out. My goal is to change the mindset of working-out by teaching how to design a workout, how to coach and how to lift. All three are connected. Designing, coaching and lifting, together form one of the secrets to fitness success – leadership. External leadership and inner leadership – being led by a coach and leading oneself. Self-leadership is a by-product of mentored leadership. Inner and outer leadership form a complex but potent dynamic to build a powerful force – passion. A **soul on fire**. True motivation. Inspiration that burns from within.

Part 1.3:
Build Using a 2nd Component

Here's an example of how I build onto the core bench press workout by adding just one more **component**, a *secondary* phase, a 3-set sequence featuring:

i. same weight,
ii. rep range of 8 min-MMF
iii. 60/MMF rest work ratio.

Components are building blocks of a workout program – the secondary components that add to the core. This additional component, illustrated in diagram 3, makes the program a 10-set chest workout. The total minimum reps is 82, but the goal is to lift over 100 actual reps.

Diagram 3

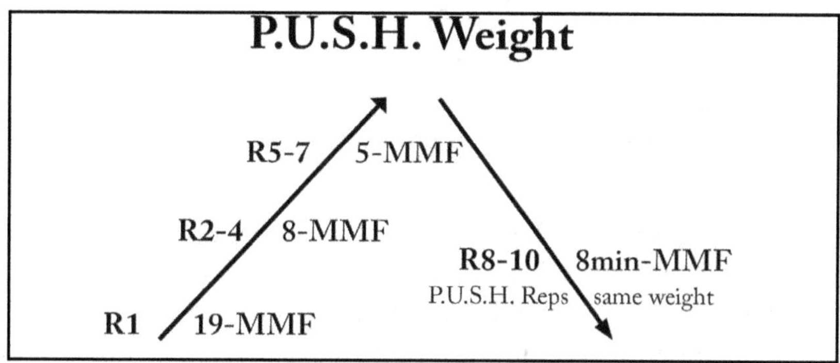

Three additional rounds/sets have been added to the core – Rounds 8, 9. & 10. These 3 additional rounds are called secondary sets...adding to the primary seven sets. The goal is to **P.U.S.H. Reps** – **P**erformance **U**nder **S**tressful **H**eavyweight <u>intended to increase reps by lifting the same weight.</u>

Key Points:

- After set #7, drop the weight down to either round 1 or round 2 weight
- Use the same weight for rounds 8-10...ultimately use 225 lbs. or 120% BW
- The rep range is 8 reps minimum to MMF
- Use the same rest-work ratio – 60/MMF...60 seconds rest between sets and a workload time period that varies with the amount of reps lifted to 100% failure.

The concept is called **P.U.S.H. Reps** because:

- Stressful heavyweight is built by fatigue – seven prior sets and short rest intervals between sets 8-10. The weight selected for sets 8-10 will feel heavier that its actually is;
- The performance objective is to push the number of reps to a higher level. This is how to reach stretch goals.

Reaching and stretching higher are natural and innate. They're built-in ready to bust-out. Goals are not created equal. There are no goals, ordinary goals, and extraordinary goals. This separates small thinking from big thinking. Super-setting... the setting of super goals – setting stretch goals, targets that seem too high and unreachable by conventional standards and common thinking. The super-setter doesn't aim inside a box of small, confined goals. The super-setter aims so far outside the box that the box disappears.

Super-setters P.U.S.H. There are two ways to P.U.S.H past limits – add weight or add reps. P.U.S.H Weight and P.U.S.H Reps are two diametrically opposed training concepts that accomplish the exact same thing – they force the body and mind to lift heavyweight. This unleashes a force of nature – H-bombs. Combustible substances – natural life-giving, life-saving hormones. For free. Safe, cost-effective legal, government-approved hormones produced miraculously by the human body. The price is hard work. Heavy low-reps or heavy high-reps each activate the switch for testosterone and growth hormone, and of course adrenaline. Heavy low-reps or heavy high-reps open the floodgates for different hormones. P.U.S.H Weight and P.U.S.H Reps take care of both. You don't need to carry a biology textbook to the gym to remember which ignition switch to flip.

P.U.S.H. Reps is not the conventional "high-rep" set . I refer to it as "high-reps" only as point-of-reference for teaching because 'high-reps' has a bad rep. So I avoid it. I've re-named it "P.U.S.H. Reps" because when you change the focus, you change the outcome. The bad-rep of high-rep is the misconception of ease; it's often confused as comfortable. It's not. High-rep is a test of fortitude – mental, physical, emotional...it tests everything you have and don't have. It's a measure of work ethic. It reveals the extent of endurance strength training – how long can you stay strong.

But, there's a relationship between bodyweight and 225 lbs. A bodyweight of 190 lbs. is the line of demarcation. Even though every level of football uses 225 lbs. to test athletes for next-level selection, there's a flaw in 225 lbs. as a weight selection – it's too challenging for a bodyweight under 190 lbs. and not challenging enough for over 190 lbs. As a solution, in addition to 225 lb. testing, I use 120% of bodyweight as the real litmus test to P.U.S.H. Reps. If you weigh less than 190 lbs., to test your "225 lbs. bench press reps," multiply your bodyweight by 1.2 to calculate the equivalent weight to use for bench press testing.

Regardless of my "120% BW" theory, because football is my principal coaching profession, my primary objective is still testing at 225 lbs. reps for bench press and squats even for non-football players. It works for any lifter who lifts for any reason – sports, occupation, or personal satisfaction. Reps at 225 lbs. is a major part the NFL and NCAA collegiate-level selection process I call "Football Darwinism." That's the number selected by the decision-makers to help select the fittest football players. I've adopted it for athletes and I call it "Athletic Darwinism." I have the evidence to prove the extraordinary benefits of 225 lbs. reps. The results of sustained 225 lbs. training are incredible.

Consequently, the goal for the secondary component (rounds/sets 8-10) of the 10-set workout is to increase bench press and squat reps at a fixed weight for the purpose of improving both 225 lbs. testing ***and*** 120% BW testing. The ultimate objective is to use 225 lbs. or 120% of bodyweight for all 3 rounds, 8-10...the same weight used for early rounds. But using 225 lbs. or 120% BW for R 8-10 will not just happen. It will not happen overnight or in a week, or a month. Don't try it as rookie. Don't be a hero. It took me years to get to that stage...years of consistent, unbroken, uninterrupted workouts to reach a level of using 225 lbs. for R8-10.

Significance of Bench Press and Squats

To reach the 225 lbs. for R8-10, I chose a 3-set same-weight bench press along with a number of other exercises from my list of **Sacred Exercises** (my basic exercises that I have used religiously for 42 years personally and to coach others).

My rationale for 10 sets of bench press is to become an expert bench-presser. **The only way to bench press better is to bench press more and harder**. Bench press is one of my primary strategies because it has consistently achieved my primary coaching goal – survival. Survival on the field, survival on the streets, survival in real-life. My research has shown a direct correlation between expert bench-pressers and expert squatters with next-level performers, those who survived and won on the field, were recruited or received some type of scholarship to university, or pro contract, got hired in law enforcement and survived the streets, or made working out a lifestyle. Became athletes.

The evidence of bench press significance and relevance has been performance – in and out of the gym. Those who have passed through the X Fitness system have made passing grades on the field, on the streets, or on their chosen playing surface. The reason is that expert bench-pressing and expert squatting build **two types of armour – body and mind.** Body armour and mental armour...the two keys for survival in any sport, any profession, any personal journey.

Nothing is more important in high-risk activity than having body and mind armour. Bench press and squats are the keys to building it. Here's some evidence:

- Winning record. Since 1985, off-season training that emphasized bench press and squats has been a primary factor in turning around 6 losing football teams, transforming every losing culture I've inherited into a winning culture. One example was the 1-9 record of my first football team. Ten months of a program that emphasized 10 sets of bench press per workout and 10 sets of squats per workout resulted in a perfect season in 1985: 10-0 undefeated record. Since "1985", not one of my teams has failed to transform from a losing culture, winning championships and recording other perfect seasons while ***playing against stronger competition***... I intentionally moved every team I have coached to stronger leagues. Although my strength & conditioning programs have evolved, the basics have remained the same – bench press and squats at the top of the list of Sacred Exercises.
- Next-level performance. Every athlete who passed through the X Fitness system and went to the next-level (i.e., university scholarship – full or partial, or pro contract) has reached expert bench-pressing level in 1RM and most importantly, 225 reps. For the purpose of my system and team goals, I have defined expert bench-presser as any of the following:
    - » 20 reps @ 225 lbs., or
    - » 300 lbs. 1RM, or
    - » 25 reps @ bodyweight, or
    - » 20 reps @ 120% bodyweight.
- Street survival. Students and police officers I have coached or trained with have all emphasized heavy bench pressing. Those who were hired and my former police colleagues I've trained with have survived a street reality involving heavy lifting that has to be experienced to be fully understood.

Not one athlete who has reached expert level has failed to dominate at the starting level before moving to the next level. This means that every expert bench presser I have coached has never failed to dominate the level that I coached at – high school, college, or semi-pro.

When at least 20% of my roster has reached close proximity to expert-level, my teams have never failed to win championships or, at minimum, go deep in the playoffs with the smallest roster in the league – I have never had a roster of more than 30 players and never had a junior varsity team feeding it. I define close proximity qualitatively, not quantitatively, as being on track to reach that potential.

Athletes in other sports including hockey and MMA have reached elite levels after reaching expert levels in bench and squat.

Bench press expertise is one of the Big 3 that has built iron-will mindset in my reality, beating huge odds, overcoming competitive imbalances to even the playing field and tilting it in our favour. I define "iron-will mindset" as a **force that moves past obstacles.** It's an unshakable belief that stops you from quitting when faced with pressure, opposition, setbacks, frustration and disappointment. Iron-will mindset is mental armour, a helmet that blocks out the negative forces so you can unleash your positive forces.

The challenge of the 10-set approach has proved to stimulate mental and physical strength exponentially. The **minimum of 82 reps** that include the built-in ten 5RM lifts has been the cornerstone of our teams' successes because winning, by any definition, is a Darwinian experience – survival of the fittest mentally and physically. Athletes have never failed to reach next-level performances on the field. And many of our athletes have used it to reach next levels of competition.

Stretching the finish line: In this 10-set example, my coaching goal is to exceed the 82 min. reps by cracking at least 100 reps during every 10-set program. The reason is stretching the finish line. A finish line is a concrete threshold of mental and physical performance and, discomfort that must be passed routinely to make it habitual. A finish line is a concrete stop sign that serves a dual-purpose – it's a goal and a limit. Reaching a concrete finish line represents a concrete achievement. Crossing breaks a limit. But, crossing a finish line is not enough – it's too abstract. After crossing one finish line, mentally paint another one and then reach it. That's the science of stretching the finish line. Build a minimum finish line, reach it, cross it, build another one, reach it, cross it.... Stretching the finish line stretches performance. This is the basic formula for achieving stretch goals. **REPS** – Routinely **E**xceeding **P**ainted **S**top-signs.

Reaching at least 100 reps with an 82-rep min. is important for two reasons:

i. It represents a minimum 18% stretch
ii. It fast-tracks expert-lifter status

An 18% stretch means the lifter reaches a challenging finish line at 82 reps, crosses it, and reaches a second finish line that requires 18% more work. The result is a stretched finish line that stretched performance significantly.

Fast-tracking expert-lifter status does not mean short-cut. It means reaching it sooner. Expert lifter is not defined by time in years or months. Experience is not created equal. One month or one year of lifting experience has a broad interpretation. One month of training could mean just showing up, going through the motions, and socializing without experiencing any physical or mental discomfort whatsoever. Or, it could mean spilling your guts. Or it could mean somewhere in between.

The quality of experience is the key to developing any kind of expertise, including lifting. Quality of experience can't be defined by time, it has to be defined by workload – actual constructive doing. Raising the bar progressively. I define quality of experience by the 40,000 rule.

The 40,000 rule. My research shows that it takes a minimum of 40,000 reps to become a natural expert bench-presser. This applies to any lift, any skill. And not just any reps. They must be meaningful reps, defined as reps connected to 5RM, as part of the "1985" chain, that gradually increase in challenge. Change and improvement are the key elements of expertise. Exactly the same level of performance will not lead to expertise. It's impossible to reach higher doing the exact same amount of workload over and over. The workload must change to reach higher– more weight or more sets, or more reps.

What is expertise? Expertise is a high-level of performance but not the highest. I define expertise as a level of performance that has 4 elements:

i. 90-10 rule. Gets the job done in the top 10%. Making it happen better than 90% of the rest.

ii. Seeing the whole board and knowing what move to make. Non-experts see only one piece of the board.

iii. Making it look easy. Turning complexity to simplicity is the mark of true expert.

iv. Passing it on. Experts can coach, teach and mentor…developing others from scratch to expert level and higher. **The purpose of expertise is to share it** – put up ladders for others. Push them, make them reach higher. Applied expertise changes the world. Expertise hidden and locked up in one's mind changes nothing.

Expertise separates you from the rest by separating from the rest. It puts you in a league of your own. Like it or not, life involves competition… for jobs, for personal relationships, for everything of value. Survival of the fittest. Those who manage fatigue better, get stronger, stay stronger, and reach their goals. Those who don't, won't. The secret to expertise is **REPS** – **R**epeatedly **E**xhibit **P**rogressive **S**trength. Use it more or lose it more.

Expertise is not the finish line though. It's not the final step. Expertise is a category of steps… infinite steps. As long as you're alive, there's more steps. Expertise is a concept, not a final destination. Experts build their own leagues, separate from other experts.

Two components (10 total sets) are demanding but you can reach a higher level by adding a third component.

Part 1.4:
Adding a 3rd Component

My evidence shows a direct relationship between high-volume and high-intensity vertical pressing (V-Press) exercises and next-level athletic and work performance. High sets of V-Press with minimum rest builds functional, competitive strength and stamina.

13-Set V-Press

Diagram 4

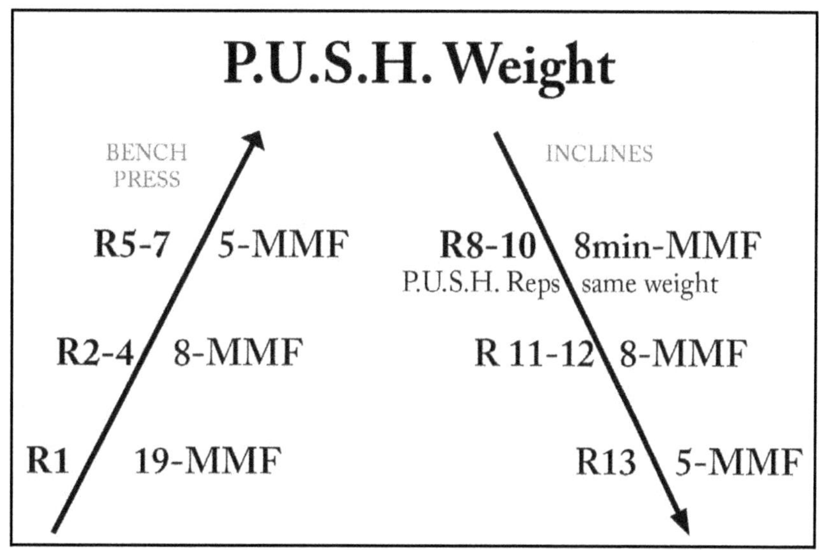

Need it – demand it. Your mind gives what you demand of it. Diagram 4 shows how to demand more of your mind by adding a 3rd component, a 3-set sequence that builds a 13-set chest program, without using supersets or mega-sets, that I call **13-set V-Press.**

In this case, I chose ***incline presses*** to complete a pure power program that has been extremely successful in off-season training for football players. I use both an Olympic bar/incline bench and Hammer Strength incline. Hammer Strength is remarkable equipment. I don't consider Hammer Strength equipment as machines. In my opinion, Hammer Strength is the closest equivalent to free weights. Obviously, it's not 100% the same as free weight but there are a number of benefits including safety and power track. You sacrifice the strength needed to balance the Olympic bar but you don't have to worry about a bar crushing you to death. The fixed track hits the muscle you're working with laser precision. And, incredibly, I have never had an injury from using Hammer Strength.

Purpose: The reason I have chosen this example of a 3-component 13-set chest program in this introduction to ***eXplode*** is because of the following evidence from my research:

- 13 sets of multi-angle vertical pressing (**V-Press**) dramatically improves striking power, an athletic skill used in every position in football. I define striking power as single or double arm extension in any of three directions - vertical, horizontal, or downward ...forward, upward, downward. Against gravity, through gravity, with gravity. Away from the ground, parallel to the ground, toward the ground.

- Striking power is an application of force… a survival skill in football and any other high-risk sport. It's impossible to survive and win in football without developing the full potential of striking force. The best examples of striking power in football include blocking, shedding blockers, tackling, and throwing.

In addition to football, striking power is a skill needed in occupations where pushing, lifting, and depositing are job requirements.

Bench press is a striking motion at a 90-degree angle, straight through gravity. Incline presses with a bar strike at 90-degrees, with the torso at a 45-degree angle to the floor. Hammer strength inclines strike at a 45-degree angle.

13-sets of V-Press have dramatically increased body armour – chest protection. In football, the chest is the focal point of contact, for delivering and receiving it, e.g., tackling – the chest is the point of impact for delivering the force, not the shoulder. The chest is often the point of contact for absorbing a tackle, or a shed to separate from a blocker, or a force to pressure a receiver off the line of scrimmage. Protection against upper-body strikes is not exclusive to football. It's part of reality in many sports and occupation. Nothing has built body armour better for my teams than 13-sets of V-Pressing. It's one of my best, proven strategies for builing functional upper body strength and minimizing injuries.

13-sets of V-Press is an extreme test of mental strength. It builds incredible work ethic, it teaches fatigue management, and it builds iron-will that prevents the biggest threat to survival… quitting in the fourth quarter – laying down during the heat of battle.

The number one objective of ***eXplode***, the X Fitness System has always been to build the connection between mental strength and physical strength by training the mind to change its perception of discomfort – convert pain to pleasure. ***Change your mindset, change the results.***

225 lbs. rep. and 1RM rep increases. 13-set V-Press has been part of every off-season program for every team I've coached and its inclusion has never failed to improve an athlete's gym and on-field performance. The best example has been max rep testing at 225. Not one athlete who committed to a program that include 13-set V-Press failed to increase 225 max reps. Over 90% increased 1RM.

Winning. The best proof has been winning. 13-set V-Press has been a part of all six of my teams' transformations from losing cultures to winning cultures. Specifically, every championship season and every perfect season has been largely attributed to increased off-season commitment to lifting and working out, using intense programs that included 13-set V-Press

Editorial #1

The 13-set V-Press is guaranteed to change mindset. It's an attitude adjustment, guaranteed to fix the worst case of bad attitude. Coaching and teaching high-risk activities has made me an expert in bad attitudes. I have seen every degree of bad attitude, every level of bad attitude, and every manifestation of bad attitude by rookies at football practice, rookies in the gym, and rookies in college law enforcement classrooms. The leading cause of a bad attitude is weakness masked by arrogance – fear of work covered by layers of false toughness. A bad attitude starts in the mind and reveals with the mouth.

Bad attitudes are poisonous for teams and the individual because the covered-up weakness spreads and endangers the team as a whole and each member. Bad attitudes are the biggest threat to team and personal safety. The unwillingness and incapacity to work hard will lead to injury through physical and mental battering by the opponent. High-risk activities are governed by Occupational Darwinism and Athletic Darwinism – survival of the fittest, non-survival of the weak. Irresponsible coaching and irresponsible leadership retains, promotes, and deepens weakness. A price has to be paid to survive any high-risk activity – physical investment, intellectual, and emotional investment. Each investment is connected. The 13-set V-Press is one example of an investment that binds each member to a team. It is one example of a binding contractual agreement to spill your guts for your teammates. **You sign the contract by working your ass off**.

There are many cures for the growing problem of bad attitudes plaguing the harmony and positive direction of a team. Each strategy has one common denominator – learning strong work ethic... a lesson that requires changing zones – from comfort to discomfort.

Comfort zones are hiding places where you can avoid any new challenges or new exertion physically or mentally. Comfort zones shelter you from all risk and uncertainty by locking you inside the safety and security of familiarity. Comfort zones are temporary pleasure points that cause you to stagnate and eventually vegetate.

Discomfort zones are the escape. They unlock what you packed away deep inside. Discomfort zones are new challenges that require exertion, physically and/or mentally. Discomfort zones are places where you have to confront risk and uncertainty – pressure points that promote growth and stretching and reaching.

The 13-set V-Press escorts you directly into the discomfort zone, away from the comfort that keeps your potential locked up. The secret to changing mindset is forcing the mind to not be set in its ways. Force the mind to *re-set*. Mind-re-set is the true secret to growth.

I emphasize mental toughness for one simple reason – complacency gets you hurt or killed. Toughening the mind needs **REPS** – **R**epeated **E**xposure to **P**ressure and **S**tress. The mind is the body's communication director, sending rapid-fire message after message, instructing the body to perform or quit. Give it your all or give up. Complacency is an I-don't-give-a-shit attitude. No one is born with complacency. It's a learned behaviour. It's developed. Complacency is a product of an unchallenged mind... a weak mind that got soft or stayed soft because no demands were made of it. Get the mind off its ass. Put the mind on notice – red alert. Instill a sense of urgency and it will respond. Not might respond… it will respond. Left unchecked, the human mind with take the path of least resistance – literally and figuratively. The solution is to condition the mind to accept resistance training – heavy, demanding resistance training – until the mind no longer resists the hard work. At that point, hard work becomes second-nature. Habitual. Quitting never enter the mind. Laying down is not an option. The mind makes performance demands on the body. The 13-set V-Press trains the mind to make extreme performance demands when it counts the most.

The only negative is using it excessively with non-expert lifters, those who have lifted under 40,000 reps. On the average, I used 13-set V-Press once a week for 4-8 week cycles to train non-expert lifters. Are 13-sets too difficult to recover from? No. I worked in a flour mill during high school, a job that required lifting and carrying 140 lbs. flour bags for 8 hours every single day – a total of 1,200 reps, a minimum of 5 consecutive days per week, sometimes 6. And, I worked out in addition to my job. Grueling manual labour taught me a valuable lesson about recovery – the body will adapt to whatever demands you impose on it. The combination of manual labour, lifting weights, and running 3-5 miles per day propelled me to a starting position in high school football and completed a radical transformation from a fat dysfunctional kid to an 18-year old rookie cop benching 300 lbs. and squatting 415 lbs. Injury free. No regression or depression. Extreme physical work that most would consider unreasonable reps… too many reps to recover from. But I did. So did everyone I worked with, ranging from teenagers to 60-year olds. Back-breaking, punishing manual labour, day in, day out. Forty hours of heavy lifting every week. The ultimate stretch goal and stretch performance. My personal best to this day is loading a 600-bag train car alone…a job that normally required three workers. Read about it in my book, Soul of a Lifter. Nothing in the gym has matched that performance. The lessons I learned were the miracle of the performance demand – no choice but to accept and meet a challenge or face ridicule and embarrassment – and the miracle of recovery – had to do it again for 8 hours the next day and the next. No rest. Fuel the body with the right food and water, then sleep 8 hours – the body will miraculously recover and re-build itself stronger than before in anticipation of more pressure, more stress…more workload. No one cooked their adrenals, no one got sick, no one got weaker. Nothing has impacted my workout and coaching philosophy more than experiencing the intensity of real-life manual labour and witnessing people like my father doing it continuously for thirty years because they had no choice – they needed it and demanded it.

How to Add 3rd Component

This example features a 3rd component of 3 single-set inclines – no supersets or mega-sets. Here are the instructions that teach how to do it:

- During a maximum of 60 seconds rest following round/set#10, select a challenging weight that allows a minimum of 8 reps. Exceed the minimum if you can. Go to MMF. Ensure the last five reps are stressful heavyweight 5RM.
- Max 60 seconds rest. You will be stronger than the last set. P.U.S.H weight by adding a weight that still allows 8 reps minimum. Stretch yourself by going past the 8 rep finish line if you can. Paint a new finish line. Go to failure.
- Max 60 seconds rest. You will be stronger than the last set. P.U.S.H weight by adding a weight that still allows 5 reps minimum. Stretch yourself by going past the 5 rep finish line if you can. Go to failure.

This 3rd component requires 21 minimum reps. The 13-set total minimum reps is 103. 100 V-Press reps has been an impact threshold in my training experience. Crossing it has been the catalyst for next-level performance.

There is no such thing as a secret formula that will work for every person in every situation. The reason is delivery – ***how the program is implemented matters***. How any program is taught and coached makes the difference because how a program is learned determines the efficiency of the program. The progression of learning is the determining factor in any success, by whatever definition is given to success.

103 reps are not created equal. This 13-set V-Press is not a starting point. It is not a Day #1 workout for someone who has never worked out. And, it's not the final product either. Diagram 4 is not the pinnacle. This 103-rep program is a transition program that I have used to bring student-athletes from rookie to expert level. Usually it takes approximately 5,000 to10,000 reps to reach this workout. Beasts are built is stages, not all at once. Meaningful experience, not unchallenging reps, are needed to reach this point. Sets that progressively challenge the lifter. "Unchallenging reps" refers to a lightweight that does not P.U.S.H. – does not include a 5RM component of stressful heavyweight. Unchallenged reps require minimal exertion. But, they do have two purposes:

i. **Building neural pathways**. Repeated motion triggers the miracle of muscle memory which leads to the miracle of automatic movement. Second-nature doing without thinking. Routine.
ii. **Slowing down the learning progression**. I call every person who works out an athlete. But not every athlete starts with the same base of will-power. Some start with the bare minimum, with the needle hovering near empty... or lower. In these cases, unchallenging reps flatten the learning curve, lowering the incline... slowing down the progression to a walk – one small step at a time – a necessary process to allow proper learning.

Challenging reps are a different breed of reps. They speed up the building process. If all the pieces fit together, a threshold will be crossed bringing you to a new level. Which leads to my **100-rep theory**. Thresholds have to be crossed consistently to get to where you want to go. When more than 50% of my team have consistently passed the 100-set V-Press per workout in the off-season, we win big. When more than half of the team consistently fails to appear for workouts, we lose big.

Case Study #1: Ironwill

In 1984, during my rookie head coach season of a dismal high school program stuck in a culture of apathy, lethargy, and sub-mediocrity, I contributed to decades of losing with another one-win season. At the end that nightmare, I expanded the membership of the original X Fitness in the basement of our house from one member to 26 – me and 25 players. For nine off-season months, a minimum 66% of my roster routinely cracked the 100-rep threshold at least once a week. The following year, we went undefeated to a 10-0 championship. All with only 25 players, an extremely small number of players, playing out of their league in a league against Goliaths – larger physically, larger roster... unbalanced competition. Our workouts balanced the playing field and tilted it in our favour.

For the next three years, we intentionally moved up to bigger, stronger competitive divisions. The minimum 66% attendance and 100-rep threshold was routinely smashed. The team won over 80% of its games. Main reason? Lifting and running. The beast was built. Mental strength, physical strength... no one ever quit in the 4th quarter. Our teams out-worked, out-ran, out-hit, out-thought everyone – off the field, then on it. A 180-degree transformation – a program steeped in tradition of losing big, transformed into winning big. Seven players advanced beyond the high school level. Two received scholarships to American universities – at a time when the idea of a Canadian on a US roster was completely foreigner. Crossing the border at that time needed more than a passport. Magnifying this accomplishment was the positions that these athletes played – skill positions that Canadians were generally not recruited to play. Both players were pioneers. And both became leaders at their respective colleges on the field and in the weight routine, creating a paradigm shift... suddenly Canadian high school football players were looked at differently. Change of mindset.

Another graduate of the team became a jiu-jitsu heavyweight world champion, after working out for a full decade at the original X Fitness where he re-defined the concept of intensity, workload, and passion.

Conclusion: Iron will build ironwill. The 100-rep V-Press concept was a major part of the transformation. Needed it, demanded it.

Part 1.5:
Derivatives

The 7-set, 10-set, and 13-set V-Press workouts explained in Diagrams 1-4 are just three examples of the how the"1985" concept applies to chest workouts. There are limitless derivatives. The following are three examples of simple derivative workouts:

- Add more single-set components. Three components are not the maximum.
- Make each component a *minimum* instead of fixed number of sets. Exceed the 7-set primary core component or the 3-set secondary components.
- Replace barbell V-Presses with dumbbell (DB) V-Press. The best dumbbell (DB) V-Presses that have worked for us are hammer-grip DB V-Presses...V-Presses with the palms facing each other. The key is the track of the DBs – the fists must push on a track that borders the torso. In other words, a track tight to the body that can end in one of two places:

  i. the DBs touching, making contact to form a triangular lift, or

  ii. a torso width – the DBs staying online, staying online on the original track until the peak of the lift.

I have used DB presses to replace either the 2nd component or the third, either on flat bench or incline.

More derivative workouts can be designed by adding same-bodypart exercises or different-bodypart exercises to form supersets or mega-sets in any or all of the three components. The following are more derivative examples:

- Add a same-bodypart exercise to form a superset in any or all components – Diagrams 5, 6 & 7.

20-Set V-Press
DIAGRAM 5

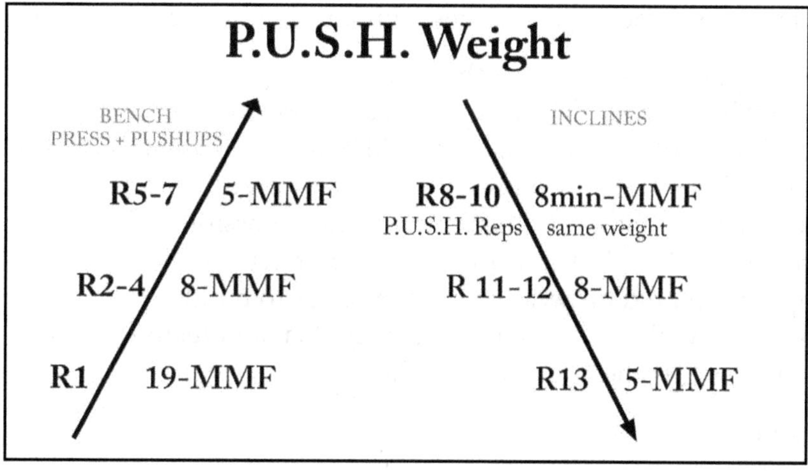

- One superset: add a chest exercise to rounds 1-7, ie: Pushups

Bodyweight exercises are an integral part of my Sacred Exercises. Pushups are presses. They are unique V-Presses that vertically press body weight with downward striking. Push-ups and bench press share arm extension but differ in body movement – the body moves in pushups but stays immobile during bench press. Pushups are a proven, safe strategy that builds chest armour, increases 225 reps, and builds fatigue management.

R1-R7 become a 2-exercise superset – 2 consecutive lifts with zero rest between. The rest-work (RW) ratio increases to about 60/80 – 60 seconds rest and about 80 seconds workload depending on the minimum set requirement. Pushups may be added to any of the components or to all three, which more than doubles the reps and workload.

13-Set V-Press
DIAGRAM 6

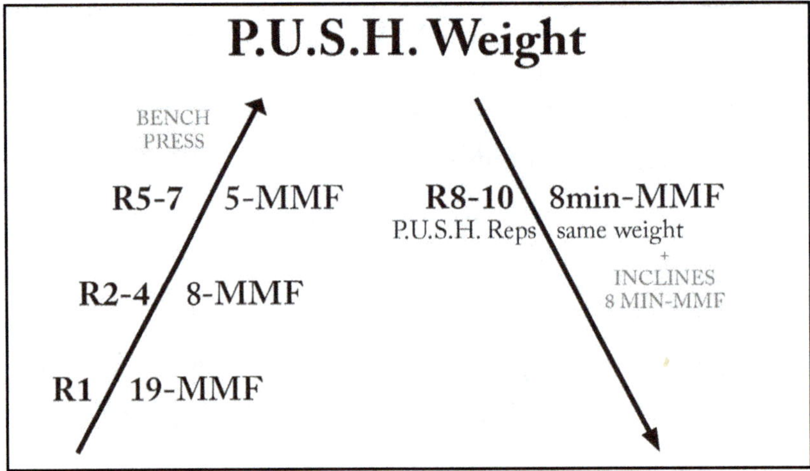

- One superset: add inclines to form R8-R10 supersets

Replace R11-13 single-set inclines with R8-10 supersets. Adding 8 min-MMF inclines using the same weight to P.U.S.H Reps achieves the 13-set V-Press more intensely and in quicker time. The RW ratio for R8-10 dramatically increases to at least 60/30, another fortest... a test of physical and mental strength that is guaranteed to cross thresholds, break limits, and stretch performance.

The purpose of this superset is to extend the bench press beyond failure and train the body and mind to work longer with no rest. Zero rest is almost impossible to achieve when you have to move from one bench to another and remove or add plates. In reality, there is some recovery time during every superset. This means the body and mind are conditioned to work with minimal rest, a crucial element needed to build a winning culture. It's impossible to beat 4th quarter fatigue without training the body and mind to work under the pressure of accumulated fatigue. The willingness and capacity to hold off weakness is the secret to building champions. The inability to overcome the onset of weakness is the biggest individual and team threat. That's when injuries happen – when weakness tilts the competitive balance.

Superset instructions:

- Put 225 lbs. on the bench press bar
- P.U.S.H. Reps - bench press until failure

- Go to incline bench. Select a weight that you can lift for 8 min reps. This process should take 15-30 seconds, about 25%-50% of the regular 60 second rest. This means you will be lifting on ¼ or ½ tank. Select the weight accordingly
- After superset #1, rest 60 seconds.

Repeat for superset #2 and #3.

Key point:

- In theory, same-bodypart supersets need some rest between the two superset exercises if you actually achieve failure on the first exercise. Set-up time for exercise number two will provide that rest. If you cannot recover after superset #1, extend the set-up time.

20-Set V-Press

Diagram 7

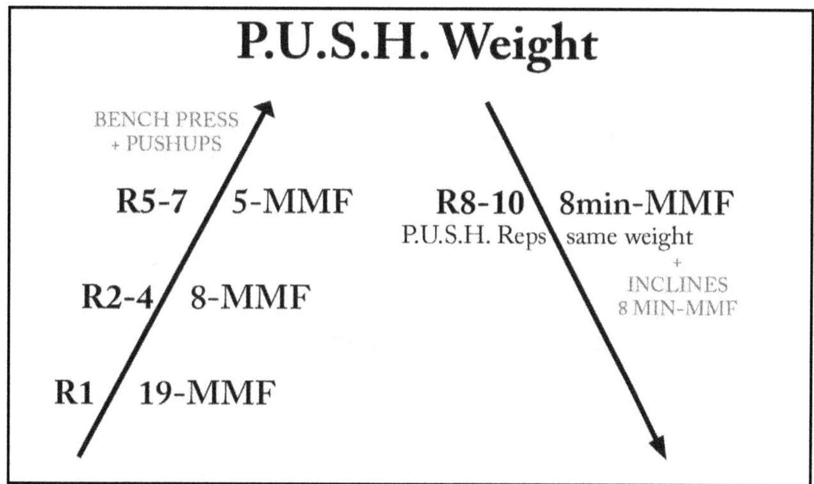

- 2 supersets: combine diagrams 5 & 6; two superset components
- R1-R7 = bench press + pushup supersets
- R8-R10 = bench press + inclines supersets

This workout features 10 rounds of 2 supersets – a 7-round superset and a 3-round superset. R1-R7 extends each bench press set with pushups to failure. The purpose is to train:

- the body to lift past bench press failure with minimal rest; and
- the mind to endure extended workload without a full 60-second recovery. This is the hardest thing for a poorly conditioned novice to develop. That's why this type of intense workout is not used for the poorly conditioned.

16-Set V-Press

Diagram 8

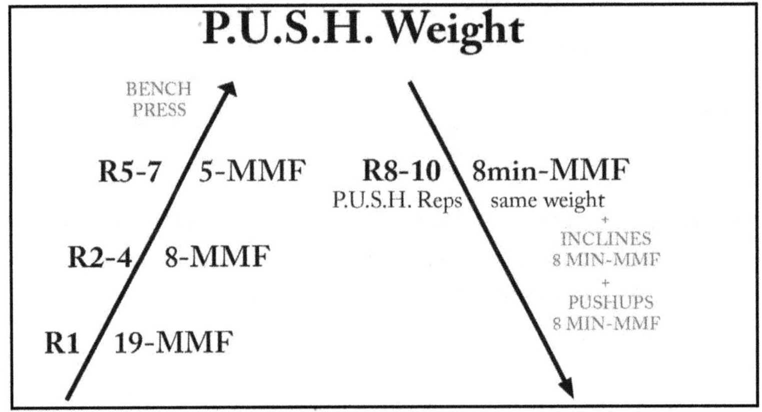

Build a same-bodypart mega-set to any component

- One mega-set: add inclines and pushups to R8-R10
- R1-R7 = stays the same – 7 single-set bench press
- R8-R10 = changes to a 3-consecutive exercise mega-set:
- Bench press+ inclines + pushups
- Total of 16 sets

Same bodypart mega-sets will need minimal rest between each set if you reach failure on sets #1 and #2.

The purpose of this mega-set is to train the mind and body to work for about one minute with minimal rest during that time. This is not aerobic training and it's not circuit training. It's endurance strength training. Extended bursts of power...sustained exertion for more than the usual 5-10 seconds. Endurance strength training is the secret to surviving any physical challenge that needs repeated application of force during 60-second time intervals. And it builds lean muscle and lean mind. Mental and physical flab melt away.

13-Set V-Press

Diagram 9

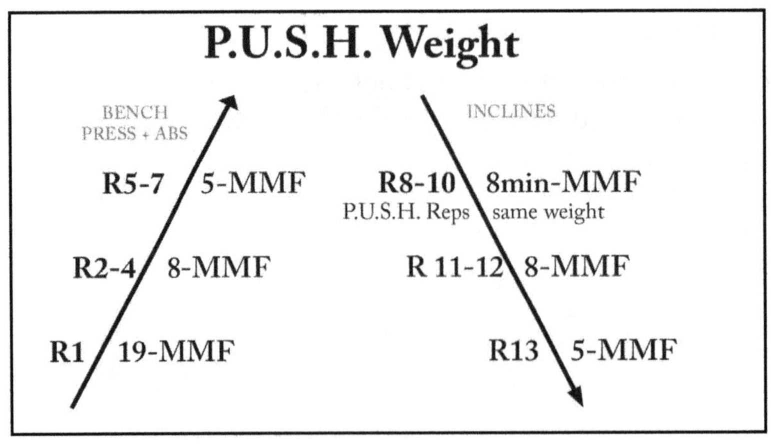

- Build a SPLIT superset: Add a different-bodypart superset to any component.
- One split superset: add abs to the first/core component.
- R1-R7 = bench press + abs superset.

A **split superset** refers to one round of two exercises for different bodyparts – a superset that does not include exercises for the same bodypart. The most fundamental split superset is any bodypart plus an ab exercise.

I use a number of ab exercises from my Scared Exercises list but the best results have been a 5-exercise ladder. A 5-step sequence that has to be climbed upward – low V-crunches, ab-curls, 75-degree crunches, high V-crunches, vertical crunches (explained later). One exercise is used per round – one step up the ladder over 5 rounds. Then, start at the bottom step for round 6.

The primary benefits of supersetting abs with bench press are:

- significantly increased the RW ratio – the workload time per set goes up, challenging work ethic. Another fortest, and
- ab time is recovery time for chest. In most workouts, I usually count abs as rest time. This alters the RW balance to 30/60 – thirty seconds of rest (reduce rest time by ab work time) and approximately 60 seconds of workload time, depending on which round you're working on and what the minimum reps are. This derivative is a total of 20 sets that includes 13 V-Presses and 7 sets of abs.

Other derivative workouts using ab supersetting include adding one ab exercise:

- to the second and/or third components in adddition to the first component, increasing ab sets to 10 or 13, or
- only the second and third components totaling six ab sets.

13-Set V-Press

Diagram 10

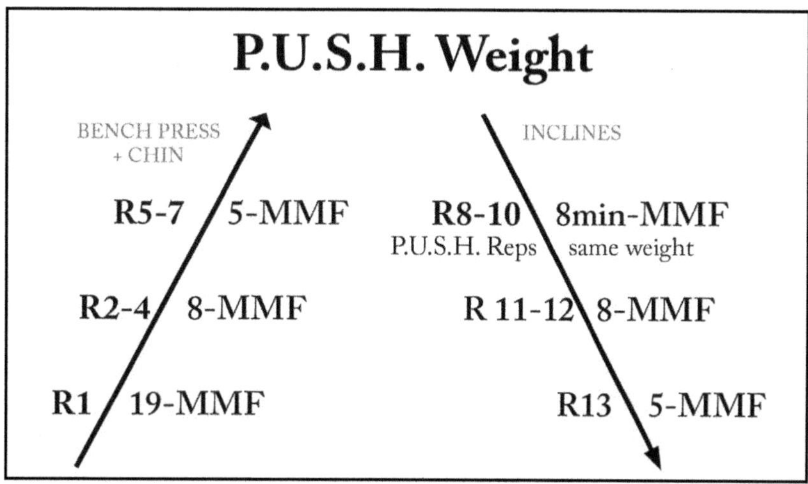

- One split superset: add chin-ups or any Scared Exercise except squats and deadlifts to any or all three components.
- R1-R7 = bench press + chins.

Bodyweight lifts (chin-ups, push-ups, dips) are amazing. They're cost efficient, safe, and powerful. This superset has proved to build remarkable physical and mental strength that has translated to 4th quarter success on the field, on the streets, and everywhere else in real-life.

I use **underhand** and **overhand** chin-ups – weighted and unweighted. There are several derivatives of both because of different hand placements. As explained later in this book, I vary the distances separating the fists for both types of chin-ups. Each different hand placement creates a different chin-up.

The first two inches of each chin-up is crucial. The first two-inch movement is called "the explosion"… the stage that sets the body in motion on its intended track. Although both types of chins require the unified, simultaneous work of both back and arms, underhand chins have the advantage of letting the arms ***muscle-you-up*** longer, referring to added arm power using the underhand grip that lets you work far past lat failure. Wide, overhand chins allow muscling-up to some degree but not to the same extent as the underhand grip.

Editorial #2

I started doing underhand chins at the age of 12. My obesity and weakness at that time prevented any meaningful chin-up reps so I started with negative reps – climbing up and lowering myself down. Eventually, my proficiency skyrocketed. What you focus on grows. Underhand chins became an obsession – everyday regardless of what bodyparts I trained.

Underhand chin-ups build tremendous back strength. Your back can become the size of an airport landing strip. They also build amazing arm strength. Biceps training gets a bad rep – false accusations. I have heard all the critics and opponents of biceps – those who call biceps "beach muscles" for reasons that mystify me. Biceps discrimination is ridiculous. Ludicrous. Imagine the folly of ignoring any bodypart intentionally. Biceps-building is an integral part of the X Fitness system because it works – strong biceps have impacted every single act of upper body strength in the gym and every single skill on the field. Biceps development builds the beast – no exception. Not one athlete I've coached who went to the next level had puny arms.

I have evidence of a direct correlation between increased arm strength and increased bench press testing at both 1RM and 225-lbs. And the psychological impact has translated to field impact – literally and figuratively. Big arms build big confidence – especially in rookies who have had their self-confidence beaten and shattered by wide ranging negativity. And yes, big arms do look good. So, to the opponents of bicep work, spare me the bullshit about "beach muscles." Check out the NFL. Look at the rolled-up sleeves. How many skinny arms do you see? Starting with the Pittsburgh Steelers offensive line of the 1970's dynasty, exposed bulging arms sends a powerful message – iron-worker. Biceps-bashing has become fashionable only to those trying to deny the truth or trying to re-invent the wheel to come up with the "Next Big Thing." Some bashers simply want to avoid the hard work associated with bicep-building.

Big biceps has been a pre-requisite on my teams. It's non-negotiable. And it works. Underarm chins are just one way to build them.

Lastly, building bicep strength builds farm-animal work ethic. The psychology of underhand chins starts with a survival belief based on the basic premise of the lift – underhand chins lift yourself up. The pulling up to a higher level fuels a unique form of self-satisfaction, literally from the upward direction…reaching higher, and because of accomplishing the heavy task of pulling up your bodyweight several times in a row to the safety of the *head-above-the-bar* position. The mind associates bringing your chin up to bar-level as a survival tactic… the head is above the surface.

Underhand chin-ups during football practice have visibly transformed mindsets. Competitive chin-ups have never failed to dramatically improve not only upper body strength but all the beast-building intangibles. I line up my team at a goal post and divide them into groups by position. In view of their peers, they chin to MMF by position for the title of chin champion. The result are always astonishing. Three phenomena happen. First, no one ever quits before failure. Every athlete regardless of shape or experience busts his ass, giving their all…emptying the tank. Secondly, the team encouragement is amazing. The energy from the rest of the team encouraging every player – rookie and veteran, friend and stranger – is a shocking display of instant unity. Team unity is my #1 goal. Strangers joining forces to form a one-directional force…a forward force that will break down, smash through, whatever obstacle you put in front of it. Workplace utopia. Evil cannot penetrate unity. I have never seen one act of immaturity during team competitive underhand chin-ups. No one laughs at last-place. No one wildly celebrates first-place. Finally, the position-winners line up to determine the champ. What happens has to be experienced to be believed. The most difficult thing to teach a team, the most important element in building unity, is instantly achieved – *being happy for someone else's success*. This single act moves the needle from self-centeredness to unselfishness faster than any pre-season on-field task. All because of competitive underhand chin-ups. Shared misery is a powerful human-bonding agent.

Two other derivatives include superset chin-ups in the second and third components, as a lead-in that connects to more back-work.

13-Set V-Press + 13-Back

Diagram 11

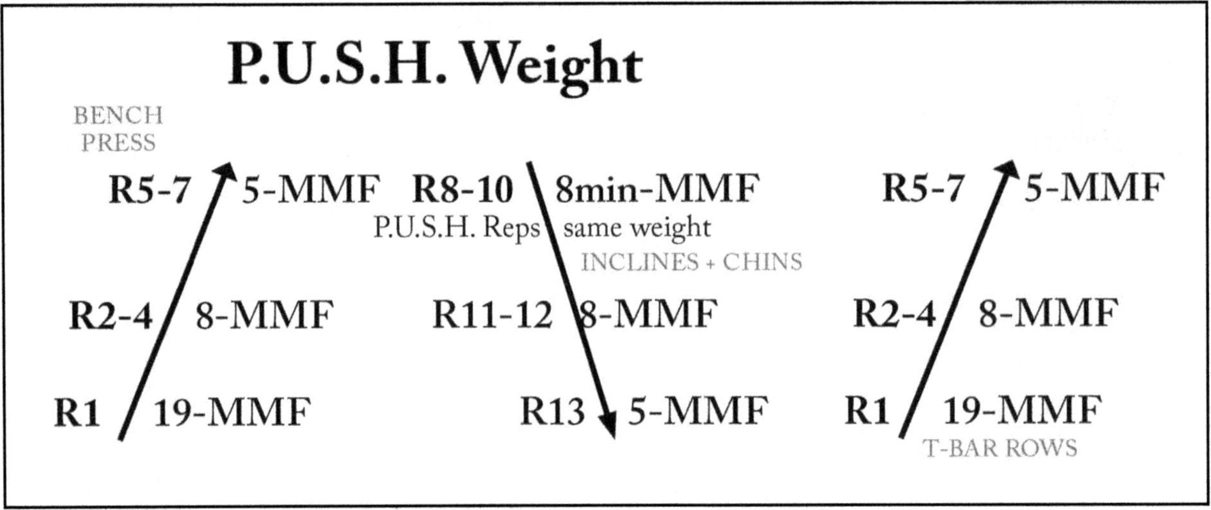

Diagram 11 shows how to connect a 26-set chest + back workout by using chins to superset components #2 & #3. Component 2 (R8-10) supersets P.U.S.H. reps bench press with chin-ups – totaling 3 sets of chin. This is followed by R11-13 supersets with inclines + chins. Three more chin sets totaling six. You can use either type of chin-up or both – one for each component.

At the conclusion of the 13-set V-Press and chin supersets, continue with back by doing 7 sets of T-bar rows using the 19-8-8-8-5-5-5 rep min-MMF range and the P.U.S.H. Weight concept. That totals 13 sets of back and 13 sets of chest. Twenty-six sets, with over 200 total minimum reps and over 200 total actual reps.

Reverse the chins and T-bar sequence. Add T-bar rows to component #2 & #3 and do chins from R1-R7.

Add a superset to the 7-rounds of T-Bar by adding chins to build a superset. For example, using underhand chins to superset with chest (R-8-13) and overhand to superset with T-bar rows.

Build a mega-set for back by adding underhand and overhand to T-bar rows from R1-R7. This builds a 21-set back workout divided into 7 rounds of 3-back exercise mega-sets as shown in diagram 12.

13-Set V-Press + 21-Back = 34 Push/Pull

Diagram 12

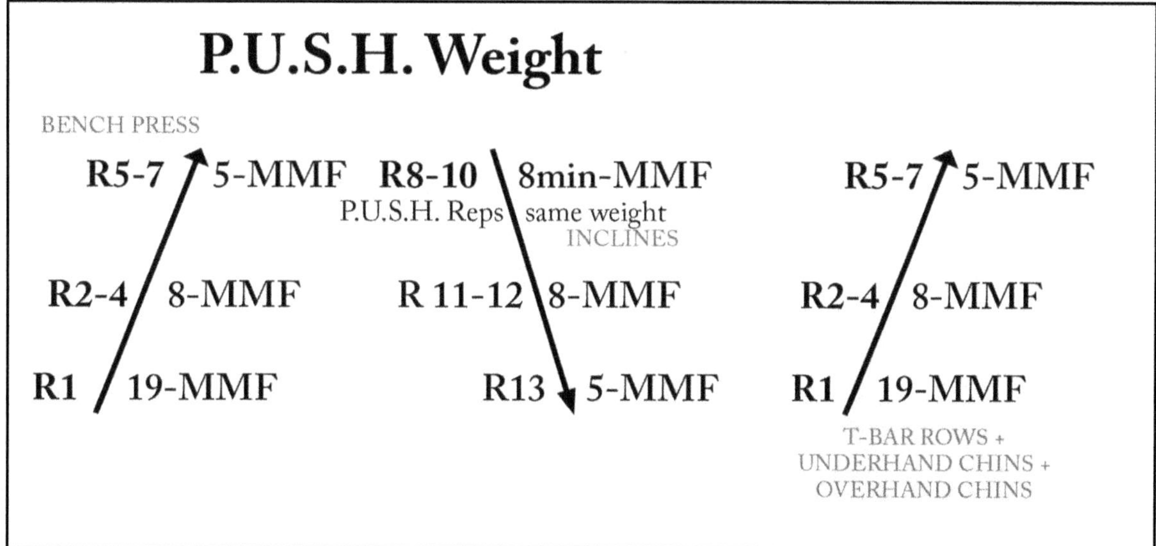

Diagram 12 shows a 34-set push-pull workout. Chest exercises **push**, back exercises **pull**. As an option, I incorporate abs to any component as a superset or mega-set. I use abs as recovery time for the bodypart I'm supersetting.

This 34-set push-pull is not for rookies. If it's too much, there are two options: (a) split it into two separate days, or (b) reduce the number of rounds to fit your strength & conditioning level.

Summary

These derivatives are just a few examples of the limitless capacity of the X Fitness system and its ability to design a general workout plan. Use the **Set-Calling©** Decision-Making Model to adapt the workout to fit your level. Strategize and improvize... general plan plus adaption. Customize your workout. Strike the balance between challenge and fitness level.

Part 2:
1985 Applied

Part 2.1:
1985 — Leg Work

13-Set Squats and Deadlifts

Diagram 13

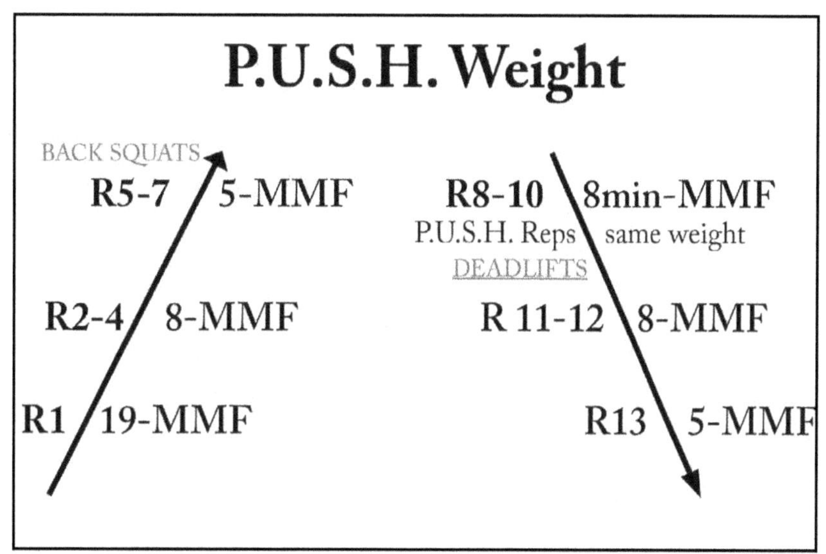

To not get pushed around, keep your feet on the ground.

Planting both feet on the ground, properly spaced in a power-stance, is the secret to not getting knocked on your ass – on the field and in real-life. You cannot protect yourself properly when you have only foot on the ground – or neither foot on the ground…literally or figuratively. I preach this to my players and to college law enforcements students – ***keep a base of power.*** Plant yourself. Get your feet on the ground from your stance and when you're moving… short, choppy steps. Don't get hit with one foot on the ground. Stick both feet on the ground. Otherwise you will get pushed around, thrown around, knocked to the ground… bullied.

Feet on the ground, ass off the ground.

There's a dual-meaning to ***feet on the ground, ass off the ground.*** It means proper stance and preferred outcome. First meaning: the best lifting exercises are when your feet are planted on the ground and your ass is off the ground because they build an immovable object. Second meaning:

these exercises result in keeping your feet on the ground and ass off the ground – preventing the embarrassment of getting knocked on your ass.

Stand up, build up.

The power-stance applies to any sport or job that involves physical exertion. Power-base refers to both the starting point, and in-progress… during the performance of whatever skill you are putting in motion to get a job done. Building your power-stance builds your power base. Working standing up builds you up so you can keep standing up.

Any exercise that plants both feet on the ground builds a power-base and power-stance. **Squats** and **deadlifts** are two examples. Pushing down on your feet to push a weight upward builds:

- speed
- lower-body strength
- core upper-body strength
- an H-bomb.

It makes you faster, harder to knock down, build body protection (armourizes the whole body) and flips the switch that ignites a T-blast. A rush of testosterone. It achieves my goal of keeping my athletes standing up.

Stay off the ground to stay off the ground.

Get off your ass to stay off your ass. The extent of your leg work determines where you end up – standing or flattened.

Diagram 13 is one example of a "1985" leg workout that has been a driving force in the transformation of weak student-athletes to powerhouses. Skinny, flabby, soft or frail, every one of my athletes who has used this 13-set leg workout consistently has:

- dominated at their current level of competition
- moved on to the next-level of competition
- built the blue-collar mindset
- radically changed his/her appearance, or
- all of the above

Instructions:

- Same as chest 13-set V-Press – 3 components, same 225 lb or 120% bodyweight goal for high reps.
- You can use one, two, or all three components depending on your strength level.
- 60 second rest
- Single-set rounds. No supersets, no megasets.
- Component 1 = 7 rounds/single-sets of back squats - P.U.S.H. weight. Add weight.
- Component 2 = 7 rounds/single-sets of back squats - P.U.S.H. reps. same weight, add reps. The goal is to reach 225 lbs. or 120% of body-weight to use on this plateau. The same phenomenon happens as with bench press… **Work-weak** – you get stronger with more work, not weaker. Work removes weakness. Contrary to popular myth, you lift better deeper in the workout. Going deep makes you go deeper. The combined effect of 7 P.U.S.H. Weight and 3

P.U.S.H. Reps has changed the prevailing mindset of **comfort testing** – ***"I'd like to test myself without all those sets."*** I've heard this from rookies who have been influenced by conventional thinking – take it easy, do a few warm-up sets, conserve energy, and miraculously a torrent of strength suddenly unleashes. It doesn't happen like that. We've experimented with ***comfort tests*** and ***fortests*** – testing following casual workloads of non-intense, unchallenging sets where the lifter is perceived to be "fresh" versus tests following challenging workloads deep in the workout. Comfort tests happen in the first quarter of a workout. Fortests happen in the 4th quarter. Overwhelmingly, the best results were the 4th quarter fortests. The best 225 lbs. test and 1RM generally have happened after an investment of significant reps. More work builds stronger tests results as opposed to weakening them.

- Component 3 = 3 rounds/single-sets of deadlifts. P.U.S.H. weight by adding weight. Two sets of 8 min-MMF reps and one set of 5 min-MMF reps.

1RM versus 225-lb squat reps:

I have tried both. For the first 16 years of my workout career, single-rep maximum lifts were my top priority for both squats and deadlifts. The main reason was the wrong reason – I became good at it. My manual labour jobs developed 1RM strength to the point where I became obsessed with 1RM personal bests for a very long time. My second priority was 225 reps. In 1985, that sequence reversed – 225-lbs. squat reps became my top priority for seven reasons:

- 225-lbs. squat reps is one of the Big 3 litmus tests used by university and professional scouts to select next-level football players. 225-reps is a major part of Football Darwinism, the natural selection of football players, a process that decides who moves on and who doesn't. More 225 squat reps, better chance of getting a scholarship and/or pro contract.

- Increased 225 squats dramatically decreased 40-yard sprint time, another of the Big 3 in the Football Darwinism. More reps at 225, more speed.

- Increased 225 squat reps increased the third of the Big 3 – 225 bench press reps. I found a 100% direct relationship between increased 225 squat reps and increased 225 bench reps. Not one athlete who increased 225 squat reps failed to increase 225 bench press reps.

- Increased team ***contact speed*** year after year. ***Contact speed*** is a different concept than 40-yard sprint time. Contact speed means the consistency of velocity at points of impact – speed at the time of collision…giving and taking impact. 40-times are non-violent speed – unchallenged, straight-line, non-contact pacifist speed. ***Increased contact speed*** means consistently faster collision velocity. Giving and taking harder hits, longer. I have never had a team that was more genetically-gifted than our competition. I have coached Davids, not Goliaths. Focusing on 225-lbs. reps has been one of the keys to beating Goliaths.

- Dramatically improved fatigue management. Higher 225 reps equal stronger minds. Most rookies entering my program cannot manage fatigue. They weaken and get tired extremely early during exertion – fatigue mismanagement. The problem has reached crisis-stage with the growing addictions to social networking and cell phones. Screen paralysis has weakened young minds and bodies at an unprecedented pace. I have never seen such out-of-shape young people. The 21st century has featured a steady decline in mental and physical toughness. The cause is work-aversion. Young people have horrible work habits. Reps at 225 changes even the worst-cases of screen paralysis. The transformation is dramatic. The evidence is my warp-speed no-huddle, an extreme fortest – a test of all guts. No-rest sprinting and hitting. Football Darwinism – survival of the fittest. We never lose that test. 225 reps combined with a demanding wind sprint program have combined to make us manage fatigue better than anyone else. Our 4th quarter strength and speed are unrivaled.

- Reduced injuries. There's been a major drop-off in injuries since we changed the focus from 1RM to 225-reps and 5RM stressful heavyweight.
- Armour. 225 reps have built bigger, leaner legs and overall physique. Cut. Chiseled. Our uniforms, on and off the field, suddenly looked better.

The most powerful positive influence in my workout career was working in a flour mill, learning the meaning of real, functional strength development. Nothing before or since has developed more lower-body and upper body strength. Nothing has compared. All my personal bests skyrocketed naturally. That's why I preach to whoever I coach, female or male, to never compromise leg work. I believe I have heard every excuse every thought of to avoid leg work or to coddle yourself. The reason why leg work promotes excuses is fear – fear of exertion and fear of discomfort. The double-barrel connection that causes the chain reaction of alibis, lies, irrationalization, enabling, and weak, skinny legs. Neglecting leg work leads to the Y… V-shape on top of a stick.

The only way to eliminate fear and excuses of leg work is **REPS** – **R**eally **E**njoy **P**erforming **S**quats. Change starts at the top. Change the focus, change the outcome. Change your attitude about squats from pain to pleasure. Feel the rush instead of distrust. Underestimating ourselves is connected to our laziness. We de-value our potential. We compromise our inner strength. We distrust our capacity and our will.

Learn to enjoy leg work one rep at a time. Don't think of the entire workout. Don't worry about the next six months of leg work. Don't focus on the big picture. Focus only on the next rep and the next set.

Calves: Here's my rule – calves supersetted for every round of leg exercise – one set of calves raises per every set of squat and deadlifts. No exceptions. No excuses. Never neglect calves. They contribute to a power base and to armour. The "I-want-to-stay-fresh-for-squat/deadlift testing" excuse doesn't work because supersetting calves with every squat and every deadlift has no negative effect whatsoever on squat or deadlift performance. In fact, it enhances it.

Standing calves are the best because both feet are planted on the ground but your ass isn't. Seated calves are in a distant second-place because your ass is on the ground but I do use them as a secondary exercise because we have a Hammer Strength Seated Calve Raise that builds remarkable strength and size.

Derivatives:

Only after a pre-requisite strength and conditioning level is reached, do I add to the workload and intensity using a number of strategies, including but not limited to:

- ***Build supersets and mega-sets with different bodyparts.***

I add Sacred Exercises for any other bodypart except chest to any or all of the 3 components of the 13-set leg work. The sequence of the supersets and mega-sets in one round is vital. Generally, squats and deadlifts are the first exercise. But, I reverse the order and do them last to train legs to work at maximum capacity under fatigue. To build susperset and mega-sets for leg work, I add partial or full concepts from the next series of diagrams – #14-19.

Multiply leg work. For maximum leg work challenge, build supersets and mega-sets with leg exercises only.

Component 1 examples:

1. Round 1-7 =

- squats + calves + standing shoulder press; or
- squats + calves + chins; or
- squats + calves + dips; or
- squats + calves + curls; or
- squats + calves + abs; or
- squats + calves + standing shoulder press + chins; or
- squats + calves + standing shoulder press + chins + abs; or
- squats + calves + dips + curls; or
- squats + calves + dips + curls + abs; or
- reverse the order of any of the above; or
- component three = same but replace squats with deadlifts.

2. Round 1-7 =

- squats + calves + deadlifts (removing component three); or
- Squats + calves + leg extensions + leg curls.

Leg extension and leg curls get a bad rep – false accusations of ineptitude. I've heard all the criticisms that they are not power-builders, etc. They do not compare or replace squats or deadlifts. But they have a purpose. Lifting a weight always has meaning. There is no lifting that is purposeless. Leg extension and leg curls are work. They add to workload. I have incorporated both in power-training programs for every athlete I have ever coached. They have three primary benefits:

- Maximum fatigue. They help empty the tank and push the limits of squatting and deadlifting when it counts most – 4th quarter;
- They add to the pump;
- They add to the mental pressure of having to deal with extended periods of exertion rather than sitting around waiting for the next set…gossiping, socializing, texting (and every other form of screen paralysis) that contributes to training decay.

My list of Sacred Exercises will explain my hardcore ideology about working out – my playbook. Here's an introduction to my legs section:

I used leg presses sporadically for the first 16 years of my workout career. I stopped. The main reason was comfort. My ass was sitting in what amounted to a recliner. Feet off the ground gets your ass put on the ground.

Front squats. Awesome. Burns out my legs and builds my core and abs better than any other exercise.

Lunges: I only use a unique on-field lunge program… unweighted and weighted - a bag-carrying exercise as part of form-running, designed to decrease 40-yard wind sprint time. I never use lunges in the gym because the on-field type are better and it gives us more time in the gym to do the major compound exercises (squats and deadlifts).

Hack squats. Outstanding results. I often use hack squats as a ***burner***, a term I use to describe an exercise that fatigues the muscle before the main event – the compound exercise (ie: squat) that forms the core of the workout. Hack squats before back squats has proved to be a fantastic strategy to increase squat performance.

Part 2.2:
1985 — Shoulders

26-Set Iron-Tripod

Diagram 14

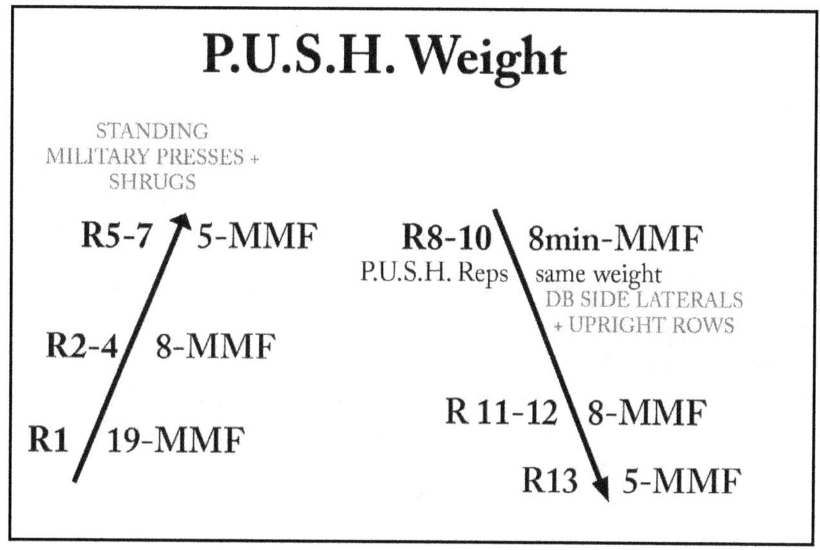

Shoulders can take much more than you think they can.

Big shoulders can handle big weight – literally and figuratively. Big shoulders are symbolic of what you put into your workouts and what you can take. I'm not referring to a beauty pageant. Big shoulders send a message... that what you press overhead is just as important as what you press off your chest and that you can take it – you can handle a lot of weight on your shoulders. You won't get crushed.

Concussions and neck injuries are a terrifying consequence of any high-risk activity that involves physical contact. Preventing the catastrophic potential of broken necks, paralysis, and the cumulative effect of concussions is my personal mission as a coach. I refuse to send any one into a world of violence with tripod weakness. I repeatedly inform my athletes that their tripod has to be made of iron to prevent knockouts, broken necks, and broken hearts. The tripod is the V-shape head-supporter – shoulders, traps, neck. Together, they form the tripod that supports our weakest asset – the head. We can't make our head more muscular, the head is an open target, and what's inside the head is the miracle of the brain, including the weakest part of the body – the mind.

That's why building a iron-tripod is non-negotiable in the X Fitness System. A weak tripod is a threat to survival in any high-risk world and a chance I refuse to take. Consequently, I work the tripod hard to turn it into iron.

Diagram 14 is one example of how it's done. I call it the 26-set iron-tripod workout. The program includes:

- 7 rounds of progressively heavier standing military press supersetted with shrugs, using the "1985" and P.U.S.H. weight concepts – add weight and reach the minimum reps of 19-8-8-8-

5-5-5 reps for both exercises – use 60 seconds rest separating rounds and no rest separating exercises. Total of 14 sets during component one.

- 3 rounds of static (same weight) standing military press supersetted with shrugs, using the P.U.S.H. reps concept – use the same weight to reach 8 minimum reps. Total of 6 sets for component #2.
- 3 rounds of a dumbbell-superset: i) side laterals, and ii) upright rows that finish with a shrug. Use 60 seconds rest separating rounds and no rest separating exercises. Total of 6 sets for component #3.
- Total sets = 26.

Standing presses: A number of shoulder exercises are included on my list of Sacred Exercises. The best are overheard presses featuring standing (as opposed to sitting… feet on the ground stops you from getting pushed around) and Olympic bar (as opposed to a Smith machine).

Standing DB presses with a Hammer grip (palms facing in) are a close second. Smith machine standing presses are in third place. Seated military presses, with an Olympic bar or seated Hammer Strength machine, is in fourth place. I change up the core component to use all of these exercises. For the last decade, I have relied heavily on seated Hammer Strength for 2 reasons: i) renewed shoulder size and strength; ii) never experienced any injury of any kind.

Editorial #3

My skepticism, in 2001 when X Fitness became a public gym, about buying Hammer Strength was quickly eliminated. Here's a personal case study as evidence. I injured my rotator-cuff throwing hundreds of passes during football practice. Every one of my Sacred Exercise that included overhead press caused agony except seated Hammer Strength military press. Not only did Hammer Strength save my shoulder from atrophying if I had to lay off overhead presses, I gained more size, strength, and definition than ever before. Note: this is not a paid commercial for Hammer Strength. It's simply the truth about my findings. Any rave reviews about Hammer Strength in this book are 100% unsolicited...and straight from the heart. My players and I have gained tremendous benefits from Hammer Strength equipment. And our X Fitness members love our Hammer Strength equipment.

Staying on Track

Hand & foot placement: Every exercise has a natural track, referring to the best route for the weight to travel to maximize strength while minimizing injury. Each track starts with a **stance** that includes the all-important **hand placement**. Stance, hand placement, and track are all connected. There's a purpose for each one. Winging it wastes time, effort, and risks injury. For barbell overhead presses, I have experimented with a number of hand placements but the best one by far is **fist-to-shoulder cap**, referring to the alignment of index-finger knuckle with the outside of the shoulder. In slang terms, this is a **close-grip**. For standing military presses, feet align with fists. Lock the legs – don't use them to lift. Don't go lower than the chin. Stop each rep at the chin momentarily – prevent bouncing and all types of momentum-builders. For the first two decades of my workout career, I used wider hand placement, but the close-grip has generated far greater power and far less shoulder pain. The same applies to seated military presses – same stance, same hand & foot placement, same track. **Staying on track** is the secret to maximizing gains and minimizing injuries. Going off-track is the physical equivalent of breaking focus. Both end up with derailment.

Shrugs and Neck Connection

REPS are the biggest threat in any high-risk venture – **R**isking **E**xtreme **P**ainful **S**hots-to-the-head. There is nothing worse than seeing your players take head shots and experiencing the aftermath. Every head shot is a brutal reminder of the importance of **REPS** - **R**einforce **E**xpected **P**layer **S**urvival. One experience is one too many. My players' heads are out of bounds for opponents. My players and students are someone's pride and joy. I never have and never will bullshit them about the reality of high-risk sports and jobs. Diminishing the potential of high-risk consequences is immoral and unethical. I communicate the same message over and over: ***"You can get messed-up, busted-up, and fucked-up very badly, so you have to work extremely hard to protect your whole body, especially the head."*** Soft training is irresponsible and dangerous. Soft training contributes to the growing delusion that reaching the next-level is possible and probable with the bare minimum of work. There is no such thing as a **stain-free championship**. Every ***real*** title is stained from what you had to pour out to win it. Every ***real*** accomplishment is stained from the evidence of hard work – sweat, dirt, blood, guts splattered all over the achievement. There is no such thing as a no-sweat, no-dirt, no-blood, no-guts championship. Unchallenged winning is the equivalent of getting marks for attendance – rewarded for just showing up. Unchallenged winning is the highest form of Performance UnDarwinism… the danger of letting the weak move ahead. The progression of the weak is unjust for the weak themselves, the profession/sport, and those who depend on the presumption of strength. Wrongful advancement is the equivalent of wrongful conviction – a social travesty. The circle of injustice – unfairness all the way around.

High-risk activities are not participation sports like T-ball where everyone is guaranteed to play after parents pay – with money. There's too much at stake. Those who play have to pay a steep price with another kind of investment – training. Hardcore training is the only way I clear my conscience. No legislation, no codes of conduct, no gentleman's agreements will ever completely eliminate head shots from the nasty world of high-risk activities. When violence is even a remote possibility, head-shot protection has to be at the top of the personal security list. Consequently, I religiously incorporate shrugs as a superset for every overhead press.

Shrugs done properly build strong, massive necks. There are three keys elements to a proper shrug:

- lock the elbows – arms hang straight beside the torso;
- lift straight up and down, contract at the highest point – no shoulder rotation; and
- CHIN UP. Point the chip upward at a 45-degree angle. CHIN UP is important for two reasons – it ensures maximum recruitment of neck muscles and it helps prevent knock-outs, concussions, and broken necks. Ethically and legally (to prevent liability) I repeat CHIN UP thousands of times every year – in-season and off-season. CHIN UP tenses the neck during shrugs, builds a huge neck, and makes neck tension second-nature.

A huge neck is the bridge to strength and health. A powerful neck is a security system – armour that protects against seeing stars and darkness. Traps arc powerful muscles. They can handle what you dish out. Never underestimate the power of mega-reps for shrugs. Load up the bar, learn to anticipate the pump. Never neglect shrugs – build the bridge.

DB side laterals:

This is not a 'finishing' exercise, it is not an 'isolation' exercise, and it is not exclusively a 'bodybuilding' exercise. It's a power exercise essential to build armour – boulder-like shoulders are vital to absorb and deliver impact. Side laterals have another major benefit – grip and forearm development. Done properly with Fat Gripz, dumbbell side laterals will build a blue-collar grip and forearms, two more essentials for high-risk survival. There is no such thing as too much grip and forearm work – they can take a lot. I have found a direct relationship between grip/forearm strength and pressing personal bests. Dramatic increases have been experienced in personal best presses (V-Presses and overhead presses) when grip and forearm reach new levels.

The key elements to proper form are:

- arms bent at 75-degrees from start to finish;
- DBs must touch during stance and after each rep – the plates must ring;
- upper body and legs rigid – zero momentum; and,

- highest point is fists even with shoulders – no higher. Arms at 90-degrees from the torso. Making a plane with the arms and shoulders ensures peak contraction. Going higher breaks the contraction plane.

DB upright rows:

This exercise will blow up your shoulder, traps, and neck. Without putting the bars down, immediately start the DB upright rows upon completion of the side lateral. The track is the key – fists have to travel along the border of the torso. Thumbs have to start on the outside of the thighs and finish at the outside of the chest. Contract the traps and CHIN UP to recruit maximum tripod muscles. As with all negative lifts, lower the bar slowly under complete control.

Derivatives:

The derivative workouts are unlimited. For example:

- Add abs to any or all the components building a high-intensity mega-set
- Mega-set with any other bodypart by joining components with the any or all components of any other bodypart "1985" graph
- Mega-set components #2 and #3 together

The possibilities are infinite. Use the **Set-Calling©** model to make proper decisions.

Part 2.3:
1985 — Back

13-Set V-Shape Lats Program

DIAGRAM 15

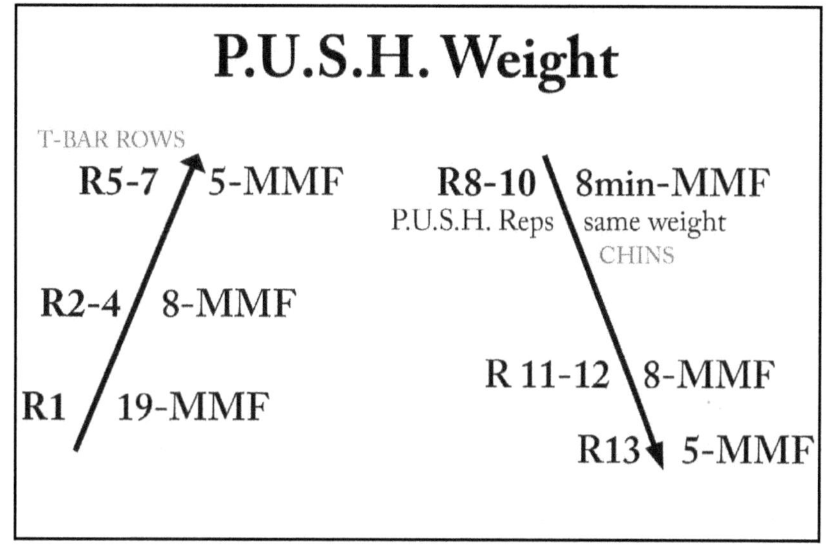

Lats are the backbone to contact sports. They are not 'bodybuilding' muscles. Although they are crucial to building a V-shape appearance, a powerful back is required for every position, every skill, and for building armour to survive every high-risk activity.

Back work involves pulling, the opposite direction of chest and shoulders presses that require pushing. Pulling engages the entire upper body – back, front, arms, and shoulders. Like pushing weight, pulling weight has a relationship with gravity. There are three directions of pulling – upward, downward, and parallel to the ground. Two vertical pulls (up and down V-pulls) and one horizontal pull (H-pulls). V-pulls work against gravity and also with gravity. Horizontals pull across gravity.

There are only 8 back exercises on my Sacred Exercises list. I stick to the basics:

- T-bar rows
- Wide overhand chins
- Close underhand chins
- DB one-arm rows
- Underhand close-grip pulldowns
- Wide-grip overhand pulldowns
- Hammer bar (palms facing in) pulldowns
- Seated rows

The 13-set V-shape workout in diagram 15 features:

- 7 T-bar rows using P.U.S.H. weight and "1985" concept;
- 3 T-bar rows using P.U.S.H. reps (same weight), 8 reps min to MMF; and
- 3 chins to 100% MMF, weighted or unweighted.

T-bar rows:

These are the best because both feet are planted on the ground, and the V-pull has to fight against gravity. Zero gravity assistance on the positive (upward) stage of the lift but full gravity assistance on the negative (downward) stage of the lift.

The best stance & track is palms facing in (hammer-grip) and fists traveling the border of the torso. The torso must be rigidly fixed at 75-degrees to the floor. Full-range of pulling, not partial. Zero momentum, not wildly bouncing and yanking.

One-arm DB rows:

The key is to form a power triangle base with the DB and both feet:

- Feet shoulder-width apart;
- Weight must align with both the back foot (same-side foot) and the front foot (opposite foot);
- Both legs bent forming 75-degree angles to the ground;
- Torso forming 75-degree angle to the ground; and
- Both feet form 45-degree angles.

Chins:

There's a science to developing chin-up skill and strength. I always start rookies with close-grip underhand to develop pulling strength. Wide-grip overhand is taught after. Many rookie lifters cannot do more than one or two chin-ups because the art of chin-ups somehow got lost in phys-ed classes. Children unable to pull up their bodyweight is a travesty. It's symbolic of the social softness and weakness that has invaded 21st century comfort.

I developed a partial-chin program for the soft and weak to develop chin-up strength. Partial-chins are done in a power-lifting cage using the side-bars. Here are the key elements:

- Bar must be at chest level;
- Both feet on the ground;
- Body at 45 degrees to the ground; and
- Pull up to the bar using lats and arms only.

This method has never failed to work. It doubles and triples real chins in 2-4 weeks.

Like every exercise, chin-up track determines efficiency. The key is motionless – the body cannot sway like a pendulum. Hand placement is crucial. I use several but the line of demarcation is the border of the torso – close-grips underhand don't cross that line outward. Wide-grip overhand grips don't cross that line inward.

The only negatives associated to chins are that your feet are off the ground, and your rotator-cuff will get mangled if you bounce like you're on a trampoline. The key is control – stop each chin at the bottom. Be momentarily motionless.

Derivatives:

There are derivative workout program stemming from the basic 13-set program, including but not limited to:

- Reversing the sequence of chins and t-bars.
- Replacing one or both with alternatives such as seated rows or pulldowns. There are two problems with these two alternatives: i) you have to sit on your ass for each; and ii) the tendency for the worst form imaginable – erratic behaviour featuring wild swinging, bouncing, and yanking…similar to symptoms of alcohol or drug-induced impairment.
- Building lat supersets and mega-sets by adding any back exercise.
- Building late supersets and mega-sets by adding any different bodypart exercise.

Use **Set-Calling©** to customize your workout to suit your fitness level.

Part 2.4:
1985 — Triceps

13-Set Triceps

Diagram 16

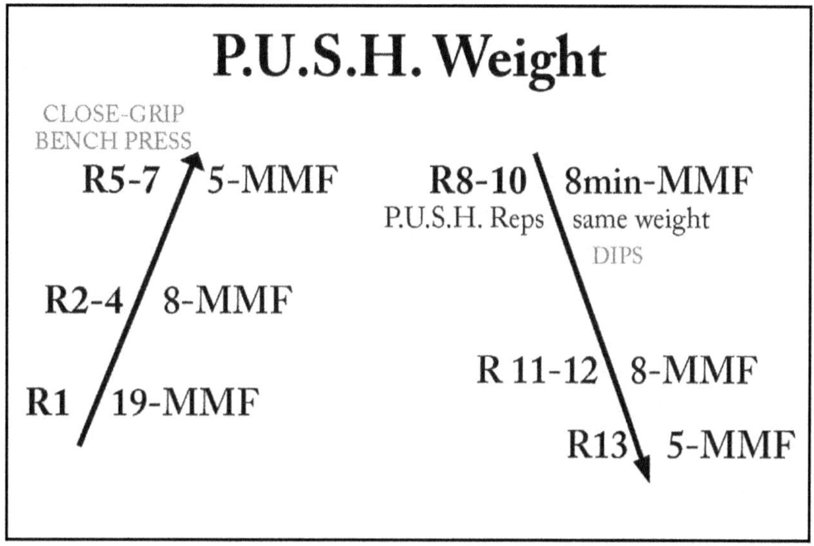

There's a skill in football called blocking that carries strong symbolism for real-life. Blockers are a security force. They provide protection services, shielding quarterbacks from the threat of hostile pass rushers hell-bent on harming him, trying to smash him to the ground with the hope of breaking his bones, breaking his spirit, and breaking his will. Blockers clear pathways so running backs can run freely toward the goal-line. Blockers unselfishly fight off pressure so their star teammates can shine. How they do this is with a striking force – two-handed jab. A close-grip bench press. Load the arms and fire – explosion. No QB is safe if his blockers have weak, puny, soft, underdeveloped triceps.

There is a direct relationship between triceps' development and strength and every football skill, every lift involving a press in any direction, and any job that needs the force of a pushing movement and arm extension. Huge triceps don't just happen. There are no shortcuts.

I use only 5 Sacred Triceps Exercises:

- Close-grip bench press
- Dips – weighted and unweighted
- Close-grip push-ups
- Cable pushdowns
- Cable Rope French press

I have removed many others for two reasons: injury and evidence – they did not prove to work as effectively as the Scared 5.

Diagram 16 illustrates one example of a basic triceps program that has helped transform my team. The program features 13 rounds/sets of the two most powerful triceps-builders – close-grip bench press and dips with a fat bar.

Component 1 features 7 sets/rounds of close-grip bench press using the "1985" P.U.S.H. weight concept and 60 seconds rest maximum.

Component 2 is a 3-set/round sequence of close-grip bench presses using P.U.S.H. reps – same weight.

Component 3 is a 3-set/round sequence of dips using 8 reps min-MMF for the first two sets and 5 min-MMF reps for the last set.

Close-grip bench press:

The key is hand placement and track. The best hand placement is six inches separation. This distance aligns the wrists with the edge of the torso, putting the most pressure on the triceps without injuring the wrists and without recruiting the chest excessively.

Dips:

The best dipping bar is a fat bar. No torso lean – stay upright. Lower the arms to form 90-degrees with the forearms. Never descend past 90-degrees. Stop momentarily at the 90-degree mark, forcing the triceps to support the body and to be the primary lifting agent.

Derivatives:

- Combine any of the Sacred 5 to form supersets or mega-sets, or
- Combine diagram 16 fully or partially with any other bodypart as a single-set addition or superset/mega-set combination.

Part 2.5:
1985 — Biceps/Forearms

13-Set Biceps/Forearms

Diagram 17

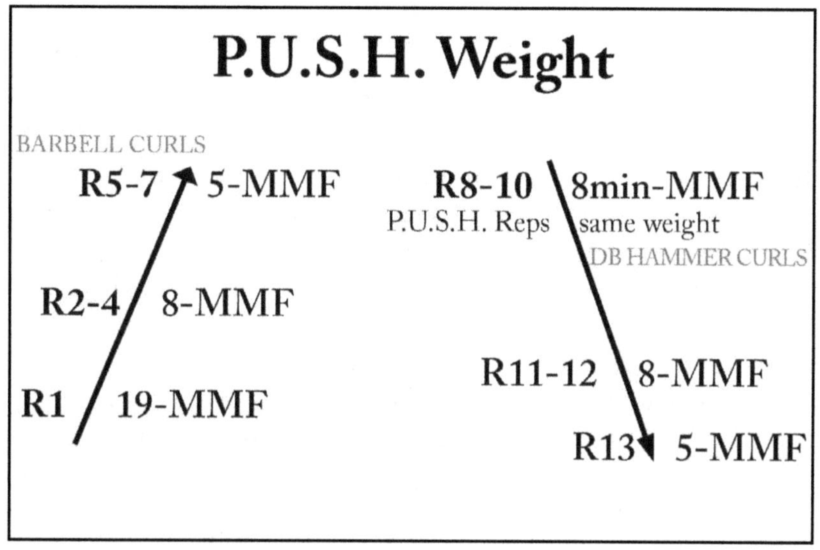

Starting in 1985, every player who dominated on the field and moved on to the next level did heavy bicep and forearm work, including the 13-set program illustrated in diagram 17. No exceptions. We dispelled any myth about biceps being "beach muscles" with the most compelling type of evidence… performance.

Here's an experiment. Imagine holding a barbell overhand in the low part of a bench press. Now, slowly lift the imaginary bar and stop at the mid-point. Pretend you're stuck, the bar is too heavy. Grip the imaginary bar as hard as possible. Look at the inside of your forearm. Now look at your biceps. They're both bulging. Conclusion: The mid-point of a press is the first place where lifters get stuck and quit before the tank is empty. The mid-point stick is a fortest, a test of physical and mental strength…the place that challenges will-power. The mid-point of any press engages a lot of muscles including the inside of the forearm and biceps. Develop both of them and you will dramatically improve your pressing performance – guaranteed. The basic 13-set biceps/forearms program is intended to do just that.

Barbell curls:

Often forgotten is the fact that barbell curls plant both feet on the ground. Any exercise that plants both feet on the ground is a value-added exercise – it works the bodypart and helps prevent you from getting your ass knocked to the ground.

Here's an experiment: stand with your feet under your shoulders. Hold an imaginary Olympic Bar with the inside of your fists touching the outside of your thighs. Keep your back and legs rigid – statue-like. Now, ***eXplode*** the bar two inches only and stop. Only two inches. Do it again and hold the imaginary bar two-inches off your thighs. First, look at your biceps. They're fully engaged. Flexed. The first two inches of any lift is the X-factor – the lift-off stage – that determines lifting success – form and number of reps. Secondly, notice the planting pressure, referring to downward energy pushing toward the bottom of your shoes, planting them firmly onto the ground. Did the planting pressure coincide with the 2-inch lift-off? If you did not feel the planting pressure, repeat the experiment but consciously plant both feet on the ground as hard as possible at the same time your 2-inch lift-off ***eXplode***s…and stop – hold that form, Stay tense. Look at your legs – they should be flexed. This does not mean use your legs to curl. It means transfer energy, a separate concept. Push down and lift-off simultaneously. Flex the whole body, not just the arms. The dual benefits are, significant reps will be added to every set, and you will be building upright power… the strength to absorb impacts and stay upright instead of getting flattened. Steam-roll instead of getting steam-rolled.

In my rookie little league football season and then again in my grade 9 freshman year, assistant football coaches taught us "how to fall down." We were taught nonsense…the art of rolling on the grounds like drunks in advanced stages of impairment. ***"Now, hit the ground and roll on the ground…"*** Self-fulfilling prophecies. These exercises built a team of crash-test dummies. One coach was a running back's dad who was a local rec-league hockey player and the other was a geography teacher who carried tobacco-stench from an ancient pipe that spread even in open-air. Neither had a relevant clue. Curls don't just build biceps. They build shock-absorbers. Any exercise that trains the body to flex from top to bottom while ***pressure planting*** feet to the ground in an upright position, has been my secret to transforming crash-test dummies into steam-rollers.

The key to maximizing barbell curls is the position of the elbow and the track. The elbow has to act as a hinge that is pasted to the torso. At liftoff, the hinge must be at mid-torso. As the lift continues upwards to its highest point, the hinge must move to the front of the torso. Never move the hinge to the back of the torso. The line of demarcation is the torso mid-point. The track is fist to shoulder. The alignment of fist to shoulder is the most powerful track. Any off-track movement increases risk of injury and diminishes strength. These rules apply to any kind of curls, barbell or dumbbell.

Hammer curls:

The best defense for a charging blocker who wants to knock you on your ass is a forearm shot to the jersey numbers simultaneous with an opposite-hand jab. Second-best is the equivalent of a close-grip bench press – a double open-handed jab. Either way, forearm work is a grueling part of my biceps program. We lift heavy until the forearms are ready to ***eXplode***. Forearms can take whatever you dish out. Until violent contact sports are banned by the government and eradicated from wo/mankind, we will continue to blast our forearms.

"Hammer" refers to palms facing in – fists form a hammer… moving up and down on a track replicating the pounding of a hammer. Hammer curls have been my best forearm-builder. It's in first place by itself at the top of the "Sacred Forearm Exercises" list. As a bonus, hammer curls build up the outside of the bicep like no other exercise. The full power of the strength and armour of biceps can't be underestimated. Those who undervalue biceps development are those unwilling or incapable of building them. Tear down what you don't have. The second bonus is a guaranteed increase in bench press, V-Presses, and any other type of overhead press.

I have been asked thousands of times, "I have 225-lb testing coming up. How do you increase reps? The first strategy is: Do hammer curls until you can no longer hold the dumbbell. The second strategy is: Bench press thousands and thousands of reps. My evidence shows a direct relationship between hammer curls and 225-lb bench press reps, 1RM, and 5RM reps. Hammer curls have never failed to transform bench press performance.

Derivatives:

Diagram 17 only shows one example, a basic 13-set program, composed of 10 sets of barbell curls and 3 sets of DB Hammer curls. Limitless derivatives can be designed including but not limited to:

- 20-set program by supersetting Hammer curls with the 10 sets of barbell curls. This advanced program has never failed to make incredible gains. I've used it for four decades, still use it, and will use it for four more decades.
- Superset biceps/forearm with triceps, forming a push-pull program.
- Superset biceps with back, forming a push-pull program.

I have supersetted or added biceps/forearms as a single-set component to every bodypart. Here's what I've found – **any combination of bodyparts works.** Conversely, no combination doesn't work. Contrary to popular myth, it does not matter what bodyparts you combine. As will be explained later in this book, I have used every possible combination during 42 years – one, two and three-bodypart workouts…and every conceivable combination of bodyparts. I've combined biceps and triceps, biceps & triceps and legs, you name the combination, I've done it and coached it. ***Here's the truth - not one combination was a failure. Not one combination has been better than the other. All that matters is how hard you work, how heavy you lift – whether you bust your balls or not. Every workout has a potential and a destiny. You reach it by going as deep down as possible, straight your guts. If you don't, the combination won't matter. What matters is iron-will mindset and iron-will performance. No excuses, no laziness, no bullshit.***

Sacred Biceps/Forearm Exercises:

- BB curls
- DB one-arm curls
- Standing cable curls with EZ bar
- Underhand chin-ups
- DB Hammer curls
- 45-lb plate hammer curls
- Reverse curls
- Wrist curls – standing 90-degree with barbell, dumbbell, or single-arm cable.

I have eliminated all seated biceps and forearm work. X Fitness has a beautiful Scott machine (seated biceps curls). It's a popular machine. People love it. I stopped using it in 1985 – it feels like I'm in a dentist's chair. And my biceps feel like they're going to tear off the bone.

I tried double cable curls (standing between 2 weight stacks and doing what amounts to a double-biceps flex). I stopped doing them because arms extended to the sides diminishes the power that can be built by normal curls.

Fat Gripz:

This is not a paid commercial for Fat Gripz. It's an unsolicited, unpaid endorsement. A friend sent me a pair of Fat Gripz to try out. Amazing results. In the past, I have used sponges, towels, plastic coil, anything to make the bar wider and thicker because the benefits of a fat grip are incredible. A thick bar doesn't just hit forearms, it blows up whatever upper body part you're training – biceps, triceps, shoulders, traps, chest, back. I had a custom-made dip bar with wide grips that blow up triceps better than any other dips I've ever done. Fat Gripz is the **equivalent of adding weight on the bar without adding plates**. And, the pump you get has to be experienced to be believed.

I now use Fat Gripz for all athletes I coach and for every upper body exercise EXCEPT OLYMPIC BAR BENCH PRESS. The reason is safety – a fat grip with forearms in the developmental stage makes bench pressing with a wide bar unsafe. As a solution, I have rookie lifters use Fat Gripz on the Hammer Strength bench press.

I also use Fat Gripz for barbell and dumbbell work – curls, hammer curls, triceps work, shoulder press, T-bar rows, chins, pull-downs, shrugs. I visibly saw a difference from the first time I used Fat Gripz. Now, I do with and without Fat Gripz in every upper body workout.

Hand placement is vitally important in every exercise. How you hold a bar and exactly where you hold it has to have a specific reason. You can't randomly position hands for safety and efficiency. Fat Grips allows the wide-range of hand placements that I teach and a 'partial wide grip' that can have explosive results.

Fat Gripz have a dual-purpose. Using them starts off as a test of forearm and grip strength and then becomes one of many solutions to correct it. The athletes I coach get first-hand evidence of their forearm/grip weakness – the result of neglect, but they also get a cure.

Fat Gripz will transform your arms.

Case Study #2: Drive

My first and only workout partner, meaning a person who I didn't directly coach… a person of equal strength physically and mentally, was a lifter named Ron. We were 18-year-old rookie cops and we worked out together, on and off, for 6 years. We graduated together from Police College. Our workouts helped us get through the 24-hour isolation of police training, at a college in the middle of nowhere.

No one would have believed our workouts. They had to be experienced. They had to be *felt.* 'Pushing past limits' was an understatement. Our workouts were epic. It's where I started my minimum-rep experiment. At the end of a biceps-triceps workout, I laid down the gauntlet – hammer curls until we can't hold the bar… until we can't do any more. The ultimate fortest – test of fortitude. The rules were simple – alternating sets until someone quit. The only rest was the other guy's set. Then we improvised the rules during the workout…**Set-Calling©**, deciding to increase the dumbbell weight with each set and announce a minimum number of reps. When we reached the 5RM level, we improvised with new rules by deciding to stay at the same weight and see who could stretch farther past 5RM. Then we improvised again with drop sets, like climbing down a ladder, gradually using lighter weight for consecutive sets trying to set a world-record for longest workload set ever.

A phenomena happened – <u>we refused to allow each other to quit.</u> We did not trash talk each other, didn't taunt each other. *We drove each other.* Instead of trying to make the other guy quit, we prevented it. *"YOU'RE NOT QUITTING! LIFT!!!"* We competed for each other, not against each other. We poured everything we had into the each other's set… to make sure the other guy drained each rep from the tank. We fought like hell to **prevent** the objective – making one guy quit.

How many total sets did we do? **Lost count.** How many total reps? **Lost count**. I can vividly remember exactly what I did during workouts 30-40 years ago. I can vividly remember what plays I called and what happened during football games 20-30 years ago. I can vividly remember exactly what happened during 911 calls over three decades ago. But I can't remember how many sets we did that day because we **<u>lost count</u>.** That's what happens when you **<u>flip the switch</u>**. Deep, burning focus…a concentration I had never felt before. Lost in what we were doing. Completely engulfed in surviving the challenge – body, mind, and soul. The catalyst was a statement made by Ron's father only 45 minutes before that workout.

Ron Sr. came downstairs to introduce himself just as our workout was about to start. Ron Sr. was also a cop. Not just an ordinary cop. Ron Sr. was a legend. He was built physically, intellectually, emotionally, spiritually. Ron Sr. was an icon, the smartest detective I would ever meet. The most professional cop I would ever work for. A gentleman with a beast-like work ethic…the most tenacious, thorough investigator I ever had the privilege to learn from. No fanfare, no strutting, no attention-seeking, no approval-addictions. The man never gave a shit about promotions. He only cared about doing his job and doing it the best way possible – emptying the tank.

Legends are not created equal. Some make a bigger impact on lives than others. Starting on that day, Ron Sr. taught me PhD-level life lessons. It started with, *"Don't ever stop working out. Protect yourself. Policing is a dangerous job. You're not a punching bag. Make sure you go home every night, not to the morgue. Pleased to meet you."* Motivation is not created equal. **What you want *might* move you but what you need *will* drive you**.

My original motivation to workout as a 12-years-old was a need to fight obesity. Then, my motivation changed – stop getting embarrassed in little league football...stop getting pushed around physically and verbally, and prepare for high school football. Ron Sr. brought my motivation to a higher "need" level – survival.

My arms never felt like what I felt that day. No puking, no vomiting, no feinting, no laying-down-on-the-floor exhaustion. Instead, an epic rush, far beyond any pump I had ever experienced. And not just a physical pump – mental, emotional, spiritual... every fiber in my body and mind.

The next day we were sore but not wrecked. We worked out again. Legs this time. And we repeated the challenge with back squats. Then we did it for chest... and then for every workout. All of this led to a 6-year era of incredible growth and 4 indelible life lessons:

- **The body can take a lot if the mind doesn't give in**. The body is miracle machine. It will become what you demand of it. The body will adapt, re-build, and re-invent itself but you have to put demands on it. The only obstacle is the mind. The mind will try like hell to stop miracles from happening.
- **Never underestimate what you can do**. Never impose limits on yourself. Never think something is too difficult to do, too heavy to lift. Never make excuses. Never believe the skeptics and critics. Listen to your heart.
- **Will-power doesn't just happen. Ironwill is built by making performance demands.** Assign yourself a job, give yourself no choice, no escape. Then make it happen. Performance demands are the secret to building iron-will mindset. It's impossible to have a long, productive workout career without iron-will mindset.
- **Unified souls of lifters are powerful forces**. We have two inner voices – one that drives us to the next level and one that drives us away from it. The true opponent is the inner voice that hammers us with thoughts of giving up just when things get tough. One way to beat our inner demons is join a TEAM – two or more souls moving in one direction. Make an impact on your team mates. Balance the exchange rate – give and take strength and energy. Lifting others lifts yourself.

Part 2.6:
1985 – Abs

5-Step Ladder

Diagram 18

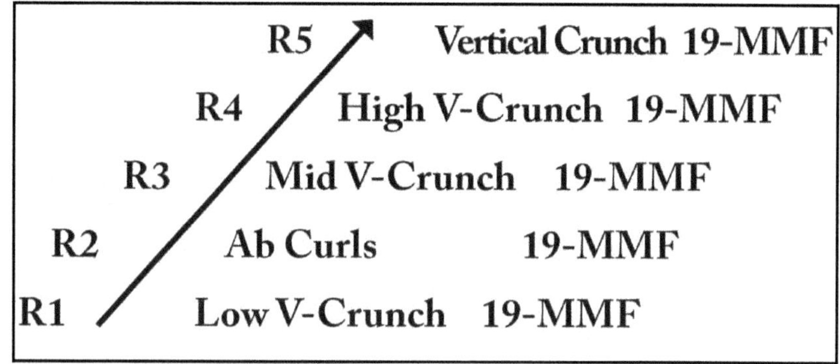

Iron Man has made the biggest impact on my teams.
Iron Man has been the secret to our championships and winning culture.
Iron Man has been made from iron.

"**Iron Man**" is a prestigious title awarded to anyone who plays the entire 60 minutes of a game. Offense, defense, and special teams. Never comes off the field. Iron Man is extinct at the elite levels – professional, university. It went out with the Fonz. But not with us. My collegiate team and high schools teams still depend on the Iron Men.

Iron Men are a special breed. They have an iron-will, armour-plated bodies, and balls of steel. It's impossible to become a true Iron Man without paying the price in the gym. Ordinary strength training and conditioning is not enough. Endurance strength training is the solution – sustained, continuous intense labour to replicate the demands of playing three times more than everyone else.

Consequently, I incorporate grueling ab work into the majority of our workouts. I follow the "Over 80" rule – abs are included in over 80% of our workouts. The reasons are:

- I experimented with 50% or less and I didn't like the feeling – soft abs,
- Intense ab work calls out the inner beast. Real ab work is a fortest – it challenges the mind to stretch itself and work through intense discomfort;
- Abs are the best way to eliminate ***down-time***. Idle time is the devil's workplace. Down-time is a fertile environment for breeding and spreading distractions, socializing, and laziness…all leading to the performance disease – broken focus. I eliminated all down-time in my football practices. Every second of practice has a physical or intellectual demand. Productivity sky-rocketed – more learned and accomplished in far less time. Shorter, more intense practices. I did the same in the gym. Reducing down-time trains the mind and body to cross thresholds. The best way to eliminate down-time is adding abs to form a superset or mega-set for every component of every bodypart. This creates active rest, recovery time for other bodyparts while doing ab work.

I have experimented with dozens of ab exercises over 42 years. You name it, I've done it and coached it. As a result, I've reduced my Sacred Ab Exercise list to five – that form a 5-step ladder. Diagram 18 shows their names from bottom to top.

Instructions:

- **Low-V crunch**. Lay on your back on a flat bench. Lift your feet and bring your knees toward you so your thighs form a 45-degree angle. Lift your shoulders off the bench, put your fists on your forehead. This is the starting point – an open V.
    - » Crunch by moving both your knees in and torso up so your elbows touch your knees. This crunch closes the V.
    - » Return to starting position – open V. Don't let your shoulders touch the bench. Head and shoulder stay off the bench – keep your abs contracted. Do a minimum of 19 reps.
- **Ab curls.** Lay on your back of a flat bench. Stretch your arms overhead and interlock your fingers. Lift your feet 6 inches. This is the starting point.
    - » Move your knees and elbows toward your abs until they touch (curl).
    - » Stretch out to original starting point. Do a minimum of 19 reps.
- **Mid-V crunch.** Same as low V crunch except lift feet higher than knees so that legs are bent to form a 75 angle.
    - » Crunch so knees touch elbows.
    - » Return to original starting position. Don't drop the feet, keep them higher than the knees. Form a 75-degree angle – no lower and no higher. Minimum 19-reps.
- **High-V crunch.** Stretch out exactly the same as ab curl starting position.
    - » Lift feet and arms, touch toes and fingertips overhead. Arms and legs straight. Point of impact is your chin so your ass lifts off the bench.
    - » Return to starting position. Minimum 19 reps.
- **Vertical crunch.** Lay on your back. Lift legs and arms vertically – straight up at 90 degrees.
    - » Touch your toes. Point of impact over abs.
    - » Return to original starting position. Minimum 19 reps.

Key points:

- All 5 exercise can be done weighted (holding dumbbells or plates) or unweighted
- The minimum is 19. Always pass it.
- Use any number of steps per superset with other bodyparts.
- If you leave abs for the end of the workout, do all five steps as a mega-set with no rest.
- Any sequence – climb up the ladder, climb down, or start in the middle. Same results regardless of the sequence.
- If your abs respond to one particular exercise, keep doing that one for the entire workout. Don't fix it if it ain't broke.

PART 3:
7X7 CONCEPT

Chest – Bench Press Partial Rookie

DIAGRAM 19

P.U.S.H. Weight

R7 7 reps – 100% MMF
R6 7 reps – 90% MMF - add weight on each set
R5 7 reps – 80% MMF
R4 7 reps – 70% MMF - rest/work ratio (RW) = 60/15
R3 7 reps – 60% MMF
R2 7 reps – 50% MMF
R1 7 reps – 40% MMF - speed 1x1

Chest – Bench Press 100% Rookie

DIAGRAM 20

P.U.S.H. Weight

R7 7 reps – 40% MMF
R6 7 reps – 35% MMF - add weight on each set
R5 7 reps – 30% MMF
R4 7 reps – 25% MMF - rest/work ratio (RW) = 60/15
R3 7 reps – 20% MMF
R2 7 reps – 15% MMF
R1 7 reps – 10% MMF - speed 1x1

The gym is the only place where failure is elusive.

Failure is easy to reach everywhere except the gym. The secret to failure outside the gym is simple – make excuses, don't prepare, don't spill your guts, give in to fear, give up when it gets too tough, don't finish the job... don't give a shit. The secret to failure in the gym is the opposite.

Failure may be the most misinterpreted word in the dictionary – it's often associated with not winning. "Not winning" has a bad rep. A case of mistaken identity. Wrongfully accused. Labeled. What conventional wisdom calls losing and failure is actually "the chain of winning." A step-by-step process that's needed to succeed. Each step is a link that teaches lessons. The alignment of 'not winning' links adds up to winning. 'Not Winning' is the investment that yields the big return, the championship rings.

Conventional wisdom often fuels myths – dangerous presumptions, unchallenged thinking that leads to blind acceptance. Until someone presents a case to believe otherwise, we accept myths... like the myths of losing and failure. Losing means not trying. Trashing your gifts, burning opportunities. Failure means emptying the tank while you're 'not winning' so that you can keep emptying the tank to win. Winning is a contest of tanks – who empties it, wins.

Winning doesn't just happen. Winning is not automatic. Winning has to be learned and earned. There's a price tag attached to winning. Full price. No sales, no discounts, no freebies. Winning can't be scrounged. Winning can't be stolen. Winning rejects moochers.

Failure on the field is too often a matter of opinion – subjective versus objective. On the field, failure is judged objectively by a scoreboard. Not scoring enough points attaches the loser label. Failure judged objectivity in the gym is the empty tank – the true inability to move a weight - MMF. But, failure is too often subjectively incorrect – a personal opinion of imagined inability to move a weight. Subjective failure leads to **concealed reps** – hidden reps... unfulfilled reps stored away and locked up deep inside waiting to be unleashed. The real challenge in the gym is winning the battle of objective versus subjective belief. You have to pass the objective test and ignore the subjective test.

It's very easy to bullshit yourself and everyone around you to pretend you've reached 100% MMF. Some of the **acting strategies** that build **false-failure** include, but are not limited to:

- Primal screams during a set.
- Slamming the weight to the ground.
- Screaming "FUUUUUCK" before or after slamming the weight.
- Flexing the afflicted bodypart.
- Any combination of #1-#4.

Acting strategies are false evidence intended to make others and yourself believe in "make-believe." It's just one example of applying the timeless rule – bullshit baffles brains. Like a staged crime scene, false-failure is intended to fabricate a false reality to hide what really happened – in the case of the gym, quitting. Acting strategies build cartoon-reality. Here's the evidence – every acting strategy needs energy. It's impossible to yell, spew profanities, crash weights, or flex with an empty tank. All acting strategies need fuel. The battery isn't dead if you have enough energy for vocal and physical outbursts. The real evidence of 100% MMF is motionless silence. An empty tank can't drive. A dead battery makes no noise.

Going to 100% failure once is a tough job. Going to failure on every set is grueling. Reaching 100% failure takes iron-will, a combination of mental toughness, physical toughness, guts, balls, a deep-rooted need to improve, and a true performance demand...no escape. Iron-will doesn't just happen. And it doesn't happen overnight. It has to be learned and developed through a structured, seamless progression that gradually moves the needle to 'E.' After doing it once, it's easier to charge and re-charge the battery several times in one workout.

Rookies

No rookie can be expected to go to 100% MMF on every set because it's a shock to the system... mentally and physically. It's a foreign place. Unchartered territory. 100% MMF is temporary exhaustion, a momentary empty tank that miraculously re-fills in a minute. But, like with all uncertainty and unfamiliarity, it's too much to handle all at once.

Rookies are not created equal. No two rookies are identical. Theoretically, every rookie has his/her own unique strength level. The term 'rookie' is a general category but there are infinite levels within the rookie category. The differences in rookie strengths and weaknesses pose the biggest coaching challenge in designing a starter workout program for an entire team. A coach's job is to strike a balance with rookies – find the right challenge. Not too hard but not too soft. Get them ready for high-risk competition without taking giant steps up the ladder.

Strength coaching has a number of challenges but none are more important than curriculum design for rookies. I never have and never will have the title of *personal trainer*. My title is coach – football coach, strength coach, life coach. I don't like the connotation, reputation, or limitations associated with the title 'personal trainer.' Coach has a deeper meaning, more substance, a broader job description, and stronger credibility.

My rookie solution starts with categorizing rookies as either 100% rookie or partial rookie. I define a 100% rookie as any person who has no recent, relevant lifting experience, meaning:

- never picked up a bar in his/her life, or
- never lifted anything heavy during alleged workout experience, or
- has not lifted anything heavy for so long that any effects of allegedly lifting heavy have vanished.

The ethos of a 100% rookie is acute weakness. A foreigner to exertion. A stranger to manual labour. A person who has never worn a blue collar. A 100% rookie has to progress to partial rookie before moving to veteran status.

A partial rookie is an inexperienced lifter with some recent, relevant lifting experience. The problem is concretely defining "some" experience because no two people have exactly the same experience, lifting or otherwise. The only way to create a starting point workout is to determine each rookie's current strength level. I use a 2-part investigation:

- interview. I take a statement to obtain a verbal narrative of the rookie's workout experience;
- physical evidence. I work out with every rookie to find the truth.

The majority of rookies lie about what they have done and can do. Statements have minimal credibility – in most cases, zero credibility. Physical evidence has the greatest evidentiary value by far. But, I continue interviewing to prevent liability. A thorough investigation of a rookie's history is imperative to CYA – cover your ass. A half-assed investigation is professionally irresponsible. Never underestimate a rookie's weakness. Never trust rookies. They will lie about your coaching, instruction, and curriculum design. Structure and records are the keys to covering your ass – lesson plans and written records of each workout.

"7X7" Concept:

After categorizing rookies, I teach one of two variations of the "7X7" concept. The 7 x7 concept is a 7-set, 7-rep workout that uses scripted, fixed-reps to gradually build up to MMF, unlike the "1985" method which is predicated on minimums. The "7X7" concept controls a rookie lifter's workload. The two "7X7" variations are called, "7X7" partial rookie and "7X7" 100% rookie.

The basic elements of "7X7" are:

- 7 sets of one exercise (exactly the same as "1985" core component);
- 7 reps per set, each set reaches a percentage of failure;
- "7X7" partial rookie includes:
    - » one 100% MMF set – the last set; and
    - » sets 1-6 go to partial failure from 40% to 90%.
- "7X7" 100% rookie includes:
    - » no 100% MMF set; and
    - » all partial failure sets ranging from 10% to 40% MMF.

"7X7" 100% rookie is preceded by <u>field workouts</u>, referring to pre-practice running and low-level resistance training… a short, intense boot-camp style workout that precedes football practice – off-season or in-season.

"7X7" partial-rookie workout:

The following are the basic components of "7X7" partial rookie workouts for each bodypart:

Chest – Bench Press (Partial Rookie)

Diagram 21

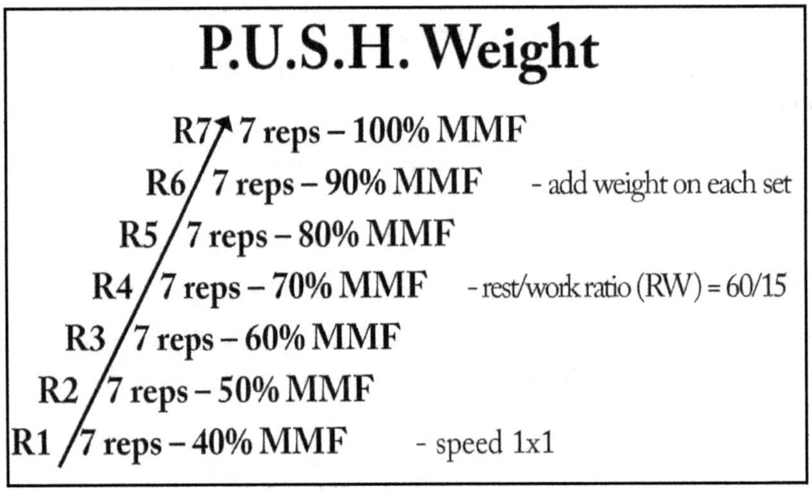

P.U.S.H. Weight

R7 7 reps – 100% MMF
R6 7 reps – 90% MMF - add weight on each set
R5 7 reps – 80% MMF
R4 7 reps – 70% MMF - rest/work ratio (RW) = 60/15
R3 7 reps – 60% MMF
R2 7 reps – 50% MMF
R1 7 reps – 40% MMF - speed 1x1

Key Points:

- Total reps = 49
- The only exercise is bench press, in this component
- rest between sets = 60 seconds
- Weight selection = needs experimentation. For the first set, select a weight that can be lifted for 7 reps to only 40% MMF. Add weight for each set, so that 10% MMF for 7 reps is added until the final set reaches 100% MMF.

The same diagram applies for every bodypart. Simply change bench press to the following Sacred Exercises:

- Back Squats (plus calves)
- Standing military presses
- T-bar rows
- Close-grip Bench presses
- Barbell curls
- Abs (seven-steps)

Starting combinations:

- Day 1: legs + triceps + biceps + abs
- Day 2: chest + shoulders (+traps) + back

Diagram 22

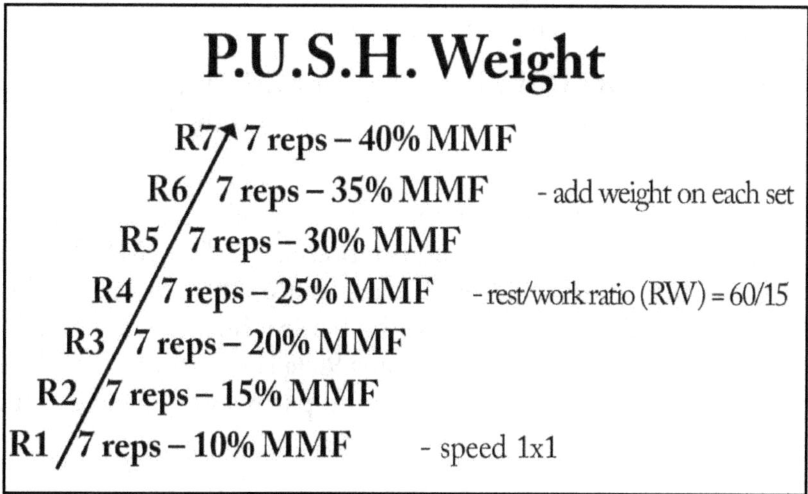

Key Points:

- Exactly the same as 100% rookie workout except the amount of weight.
- Use weight that ranges from only 10% - 40% MMF, increasing by 5% increments.
- 100% rookie field workouts: Before working out in the gym, 100% rookies do the following workout.

5-Stage Form Running:

- stage 1 – 3 sets of unweighted forward lunges,
- stage 2 – 3 sets of unwieghted side lunges,
- stage 3 – 3 sets of 5 yard high-step sprint (six inch strides),
- stage 4 – 3 sets of 40-yard long-stride sprint,
- stage 5 – 3 sets of 10-yard sprint form stance to 45-degree torso lean
- 3 sets of 40-yard bear crawl sprints
- 3 sets of 20 chest pushups (thumbs align with shoulder cap)
- 3 sets of 20 close-grip pushups (thumbs and index fingers form a triangle)
- 3 sets of underhand chins on the goal-posts
- 3 sets of over-hand chins on the goal-posts
- 3 sets of bag-carrying – sprint 40 yards with tackling dummy on shoulder
- 3 sets of front squats – holding tackling dummy
- 3 sets of tractor tire deadlift
- 3 sets of tractor tire plyometrics
- 12 sets of blocking sled – using a 7-man sled: 4 sets x 7-man, 4 sets x 5-man, 4 sets x 3-man

The field workout has transformed form and fitness in 5-10 days. I use the same field workout to start every practice, in-season or off-season. The benefits are immeasurable. This program has been the backbone of on-field and gym successes.

What exactly is a percentage of MMF? Percentage of MMF is an abstract concept. The objective is to convert each MMF percentage to concrete weight on the bar. The way to do it is find a point-of-reference.

The best point of reference is the bar with no weight. Any of the "7X7" Sacred Exercises can be performed with just the bar. A bar without weight represents 10% MMF. This may seem incredibly light but it isn't for a 100% rookie. Never underestimate 100% rookie weakness. Trying to make a 100% rookie into an action hero right off the bat is a horrible mistake. Resist the temptation to "prove how tough you are." 10% MMF means 90% is left in the tank. The main purpose of 10% MMF is learning proper form and building neural pathways – muscle memory. Automatic second-nature lifts.

The next important point-of-reference is the struggle-point. The percentage of a set that requires a struggle corresponds with percentage of MMF:

- 50% MMF requires no struggle for the entire set
- 75% MMF requires struggle for the last 25% of the set
- 100% MMF requires struggle for the last 50% of the set

Rule: The percentage of struggle per set corresponds with percentage of MMF. Zero struggle corresponds with 10%-50% MMF. After 50% MMF, the percentage of struggle directly corresponds with %MMF. The maximum struggle to reach 100% MMF for 7 reps is 50% struggle. 50% is the line of demarcation. If struggle happens before the 50% line, the weight is too heavy for 7 reps.

I define "struggle" as contested lifting – a level of exertion that exceeds ease. Struggle happens when the level of resistance demands maximum recruitment of muscle fibers. Uncontested lifting is not a struggle. Non-struggle occurs when the resistance is less than the strength. Non-struggle happens when: (a) the weight is too light, or (b) the weight is heavy enough but fatigue has not affected the lift.

Overcoming struggle is a learned skill. It doesn't just happen. It has to be built – incrementally. The "7X7" concept has been my best strategy for building the inner beast.

Rationale for 7 reps for 7 sets

Why was "7X7" chosen? Best practice.

Everything I teach and how I teach it is the product of the Best Practices Model that I designed in my M.Ed. thesis:

Best Practice Model

Diagram 23

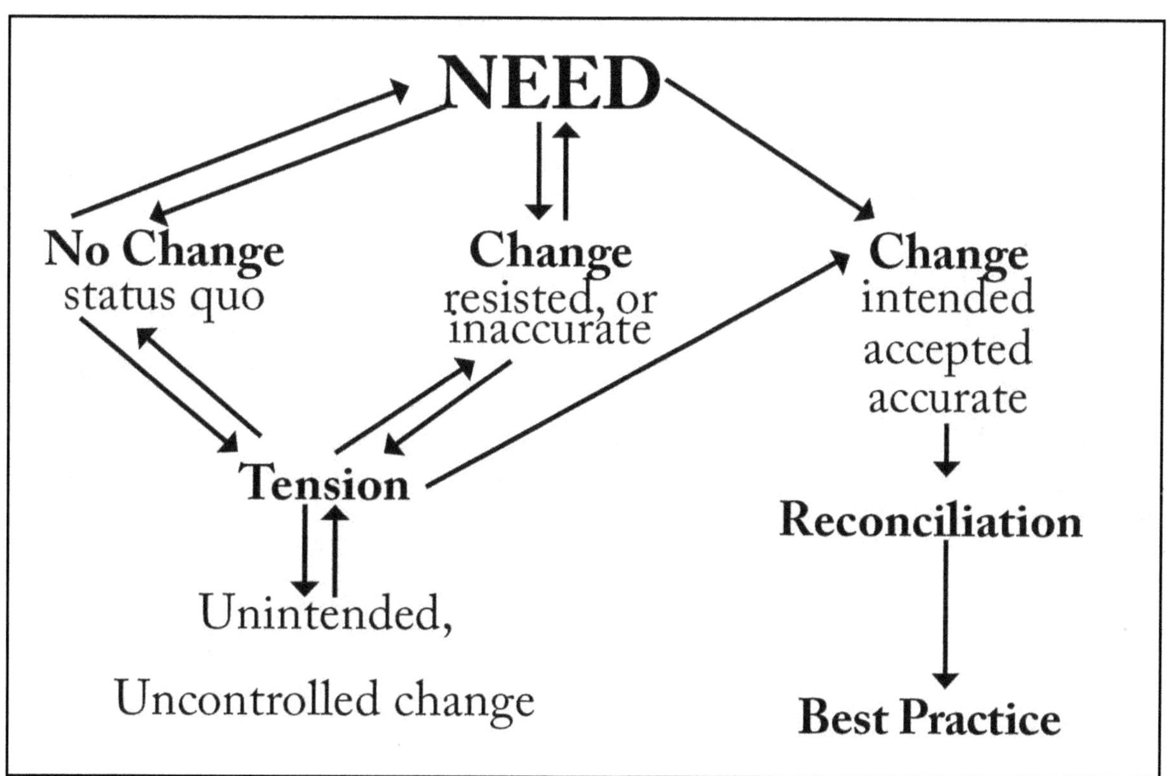

This chart is an investigative model intended to solve problems. I have used this chart to design curriculum, teaching strategies, and testing for football, college law enforcement, and strength training. And, I used it to solve crimes.

The basic theory behind this model is that there is a solution, called a Best Practice, to any mystery, referring to the best strategy to achieve a specific goal. But, Best Practices have to be discovered. Discoveries are the product of proactive experimentation. Making it happen as opposed to waiting for it to happen. The secret to proactive experimentation is structured testing – not random winging it. Every profession I've worked in taught me the value of proactive experimentation – how to test a theory to determine what works and what doesn't in my teams' specific reality.

Of all the programs I have tested for rookies, "7X7" has worked the best at transforming physical strength, appearance, and mindset. How? By changing work ethic and making working out a basic survival need. The total of **147 reps** spread over 21 sets for three bodyparts separated by a maximum of 60 seconds rest has outgained any other workout combination that I have tested. The workout usually takes less than 30 minutes – 21 minutes of rest and about 5 minutes of total workload. The rest/work ratio per set is 60/14. Sixty seconds rest and 14 seconds of lifting (1x1 speed for 7 reps).

"7X7" derivatives:

Add or subtract sets and/or reps, using the **Set-Calling©** model. As stated, rookies are not created equal… neither is their progress. Rookie commitment is erratic. Failing to appear for workouts is a rookie reality that blocks progress. Showing up is the most important part of rookie training. Those who do, progress. Those who don't, regress.

One of the best derivatives is a 2-bodypart 10x10 P.U.S.H. Reps – 10 sets of 10 min reps using exactly the same weight. It can be used as a superset with less than 60 seconds rest or single-set with 30-60 seconds rest. I have tried every combination of double bodyparts with equal effects. No combination has been better or worse. What matters is the effort invested, not the combination of bodyparts.

"7X7" for veteran lifters:

Generally, I work out 26 out of 28 days. I never take extended time off. I cannot remember that last time I took a week off. Taking two days off is a rarity because after one day off, I start to suffer mentally and physically. I use the "7X7" concept, or a derivative, as an active rest from the more grueling concepts in the ***eXplode*** System that call for 100% MMF, like "1985". Depending on how much recovery I need, I generally use "7X7" for 1-2 weeks after a prolonged intense workout stage. "7X7" is a back-to-the-basics break from megaset workouts.Ad ditionally, I sometimes incorporate "7X7" concepts for in-season workouts. It's incredibly effective for players to supplement their field workouts and for myself when work and coaching create serious time constraints.

Case Study #3: Losing Your SUAL

"What set are we on?" There are only two causes for asking that question – intense focus or no focus.

Intense focus can make you lose count by losing yourself – full immersion in a workout that blocks out everything except what has to be done in the moment. Losing yourself is a rare state of mind where you go deeper than you thought you could go to find and release new sources of energy – self-discovery of power sources – a process that takes every mental fiber. Maximum mental fiber recruitment. When every mental fiber is preoccupied, you lose count…and you call out the inner beast. That's the true power of focus.

No focus has the same effect of losing count. No focus is a growing social problem. It happens when you **lose your SUAL** – when you lose the ability to Shut Up And Lift. Between 1985-2000, I never had problems with my teams' workout focus. They were silent warriors – they knew how to Shut Up And Lift. They understood the Iron Rule the first time they learned it – the sanctity of the gym demands silence – never lose your SUAL. They saw the evidence of the power of SUAL – high-performance. They understood the reason for a healthy SUAL – unwavering focus. Concentration is connected to performance. Laser-like focus is the catalyst for calling out the inner beast. Broken focus gets you knocked down by the outer beasts.

SUAL never failed to achieve incredible results. Workouts were memorable experiences. Some players described them as spiritual experience 25 years later. Then something happened – the 21st century. Socializing – the focus-breaker. Nothing destroys concentration quicker than idle chatter and meaningless conversation – bar talk instead of bar lifting.

Social networking spilled over into the gym. My coaching job description grew to include "day-care supervisor." Constantly reminding people to SUAL is the biggest distraction to my own workouts. Addictions to socializing prevent people of all ages from putting their minds to lifting for what amounts to a very small percentage of their day. The addiction has spread to everyone I coach – male or female, younger or older, competitive athlete or non-competitive athlete – all drain me faster than a set of heavy squats. Constantly reminding people to SUAL is compelling evidence of one the most powerful fears that hold us back – fear of isolation. The fear of not being connected socially every moment. It's the #1 reason why fitness goals are not met. It's the leading cause of procrastination, not finishing a job, not giving it your all, not sticking to a mission, quitting.

Quitting is the by-product of the Chain of Fear. Fear of isolation is linked with the fear of discomfort…the pain of physically and/or mentally stretching. If the Chain of Fear is not broken, quitting is inevitable. The mind will invent every excuse possible to rationalize quitting – not enough time, not enough money, not enough freedom, not enough shiny machines…no excuse is too far-fetched. The mind will make-up make-believe and make you believe it. That's the ethos of the untrained mind – the lost SUAL.

In June, 2011, I was training a team of partial rookies – female and male. Even though each individual had been working out for more than one year, they were still rookies. Each one asked me to coach them – I didn't ask them. Their decision to get coached by me must be voluntary, meaning the product of self-generated inducement. Inner inducement. That's my non-negotiable philosophy. I used this strategy to attract students to college also. Instead of selling and recruiting I inform people of our existence, our track record, and the *opportunity to grow.* Then I let free will get exercised.

As usual, I worked out with the group. I coach actively in the gym, not passively. Because of the numbers, I divided the group into two, to prevent zero down-time, and gave the first group my "7X7" instructions. The second group was nearby, not miles away, not on a different floor. Close proximity. But far enough for the socializing to escalate. After 5 minutes, I heard the evidence of broken focus: *"What set are we on?"*

A coaching moment. *It's impossible to release your potential while you're opposing it. Resistance to full-focus resistance training has to be eliminated from within.* **Full-focus, full-force.** Both impossible without SUAL.

Case Study #4: F-Bombing a Set

"FUUUUCK!!!"

On the fourth set of a 5-mininum bench press, one of my athlete-clients e**X**ploded an F-Bomb like he had just realized the price of gas. The 5th set failed. Dropped to his chest. The wrong kind of failure.

A coaching moment. *The energy wasted to e**X**plode an F-bomb wasted reps. Hid them. Locked them up. Threw them onto the growing heap of concealed reps that you're carrying around like a heavy weight.*

And, the weight was light for a guy who allegedly has worked out for three years. This was an embarrassment for a guy in his mid-20's who desperately wants a uniform and badge – to enter the dark side of society – and fight evil. Save your F-Bombs, don't save your reps.

The failed 5th rep was evidence of "1985" weakness. Incapable of playing in the big leagues. He was demoted to partial rookie status. Back to "7X7". That's how the system works.

Case Study #5: Confucktions

Born weak, stay weak. That's what the mind wants to achieve. The toughest part of working out, bar none, is conquering the mind and its' whining, complaining dialogue that pollutes first our thoughts and then the air around us. I invented a word for the cause of this – confucktion. A confucktion is a malfunction that fucks up logic. Confucktions have a distinct sound – rationalizing irrationality.

Since 2006, one of my former college students has asked me for advice ranging from how to pass police testing, how to answer job interview questions, how to build muscle, and how to "get mentally tougher." Without ever asking the cost (the presumption of charity). What he was asking for was a complete makeover – mental, physical, and life. If he went to a psychiatrist or psychologist, his therapy bill would have been astronomical. But he presumed that fitness credibility is applicable only to non-profit organizations, a presumption that I had been guilty of promoting, unfortunately.

For those who are or aspire to become fitness coaches, here's some advice – don't do what I've done. Never de-value yourself. Never build yourself a bad rep…a reputation of donating your expertise and time for free. I have never been paid a cent for coaching football, the same job that many coaches earn annual salaries in the 3-million dollar range. During my coaching time, I have given away strength, employment, and life coaching for free to those same athletes. Conservatively, if I had been paid minimum wage for all my coaching hours that I have given away – on the field, in the gym, in the counseling office – I would have earned $1.2 million dollars …Canadian.

On the fourth day after he got his uniform, this same student asked for help. It turns out he got weak from laying off working out, saw the real-life up close and personal, got scared that he couldn't cut it and would get bounced around the streets, and asked for strength coaching. Week one revealed the weak one. Four years of alleged workout experience got him demoted to partial rookie. Week four revealed a weaker one – he missed 5 out of six days because his "girlfriend couldn't understand why working out so much is necessary. She thought once a week was enough." Upon his return to the gym, he complained, out-loud during a hammer curl set, while I corrected his form. After he put down the dumbbells, he announced, "This is hard!"

A coaching moment . *Don't blame me for your weakness.* I fired him. In the past, I would have stuck it out until I cured his confucktions. I fought to fix the broken because I believed I could save the world. Not anymore. I refuse to enable weakness. Chronic confucktions have to be cured from the inside. Any opportunity to grow is sacred. The most important fitness is the proper exercise of free will. Trashing an opportunity cannot be rewarded.

Opportunities are a matter of perception. A weak mind sees a chance to back out and quit. A strong mind sees a challenge. A weak mind rationalizes irrationalization. A strong mind accepts responsibility. A weak mind sees a curse. A strong mind sees a blessing.

Case Study #6: I Saw A Miracle This Week

Actually, two. I saw two miracles this week – the first week of July, 2011. My granddaughter Violet is 11 months old. Yesterday, she walked up to my 5 lb. barrel of protein powder. She grabbed the handle and deadlifted it. The barrel was empty but heavy is relative. On her second rep, she broke out in the biggest smile I have ever witnessed in my life. And she kept smiling during her 3rd rep and 4th rep and 5th rep.

For her second set, she pushed the barrel like a blocking sled, driving it across the floor for 10 yards, cheering herself on. Her third set was the toughest – upright rows. Four reps. Strict form, no cheating. Under control, she put the weight back on floor. She didn't slam it, drop it, or smash it to the ground. No, she put the barrel down under control. Even an infant knows the positives of the negative rep – lower the weight under control, don't slam it to the ground endangering yourself and everyone around you.

Then, the adrenaline rush. Clapping her hands, waving her arms…the baby pump, that magical feeling when the switch goes on and all is well in the world.

Thirty minutes later, we went to the park. I witnessed another miracle. Violet sprinted the equivalent of two football fields. Smiling, cheering, waving wildly… poor arm form, questionable stride length but here's the miracle part – she never quit. Never made excuses. Never whined, never complained. Never mouthed off, no intolerable attitude. No sense of entitlement, not a hint of laziness. She finished her wind sprints happier than when she started them.

I have been blessed to have coached thousands of student-athletes, blessed to have taught thousands of wannabe cops, blessed to have seen some amazing performances but I have never seen anything like Violet's workout. Less than one year on planet Earth and already passionate above lifting and running. I thank God Almighty for the miracle of cell phone cameras so I can replay it over and over and over. Reps of pure joy.

I have devoted my entire adult life to urging other peoples' children to lift and run and play hard. I have pleaded with them to not waste their gifts…to unleash everything they have, to not bury their talents. And I have pleaded with them to love it…pleaded with them to embrace their blessings of great health and to love lifting and love running and love playing hard together. Some listened, some didn't.

I'm still dedicating my life to those things but now I'm adding one more – I'm devoting every ounce of energy I've got to make sure that Violet never loses her passion for lifting hard and running hard, never stops smiling, laughing, and waving her arms wildly, never buries her gifts and talents, never falls under the influence of gloom, doom, and negativity, and most of all…never loses her soul of a lifter.

Keep lifting Violet… lift as many souls as you can, every minute, every day. Never stop lifting, Violet.

Case Study #7: Turning Back the Clock

On July 25, 2011, I turned 54. I celebrated using my **Set-Calling©** principals with a 43-set, 652-rep leg and abs workout, followed by a 45-minute run that included 10 wind sprints at the end.

The next day, I celebrated my 54th birthday with a 40-set, 458-rep chest, traps, and abs workout followed by another 45 minute run and 8 wind sprints at the end.

The next day, I celebrated my 54th birthday with a 40-set, 444-rep back and shoulder workout followed by another 45-minute run and 8 wind sprints.

The next day, I celebrated my 54th birthday with a 44-set, 728-reps triceps, biceps, forearms, and abs workout followed by another 45-minute run and 10 wind sprints.

My wife is a witness. But witness statements are susceptible to poor credibility. Physical evidence has the higher value. Each one of these workouts is on film, electronically recorded and archived by the 24-hour security cameras inside X Fitness – videotape of every rep that is lifted during every 24-hour workday.

I divide my workouts into 4-quarter programs. My birthday celebration was the 4th quarter of phase 10 of my current one-year program.

Why do I do this? Two reasons. First, fear of becoming obese like I was at 12 years old. I fight fat every day of my life. I've experienced obesity, overcame it, and I refuse to live the only life I will have on planet Earth with mounds of blubber hanging and banging with every move I make. Secondly, fear of being like most people I've known – become a senior citizen at age 30, start wearing cardigans, ask for 15% discounts, be a martyr by posting your ailments and misfortunes for the whole world to read on Facebook, re-live glory days on the 19th hole, live vicariously through your children, through dancing stars, through singing idols, and through immature megalomaniacs who get paid millions to play kids games.

I turned back the clock by the combined effect of working out for 42 years and escaping soul-killing workplaces. Becoming a full-time business owner, writer, football coach, and full-time athlete is the smartest, healthiest decision I've made. Working out is my career, not a hobby. I've made it a basic survival need. I need it to test myself every day. I need it to self-actualize, to reveal every physical and mental fiber of my potential. I need the physical pump, the intellectual pump, the emotional pump, but most importantly, I need to get the spiritual pump.

This ends Part 3 – the introduction – teaching only two workout concepts and the basic philosophy and psychology of *eXplode*, the X Fitness System. Part 4 explains the system in greater detail.

∞

Part 4: The X Factor System

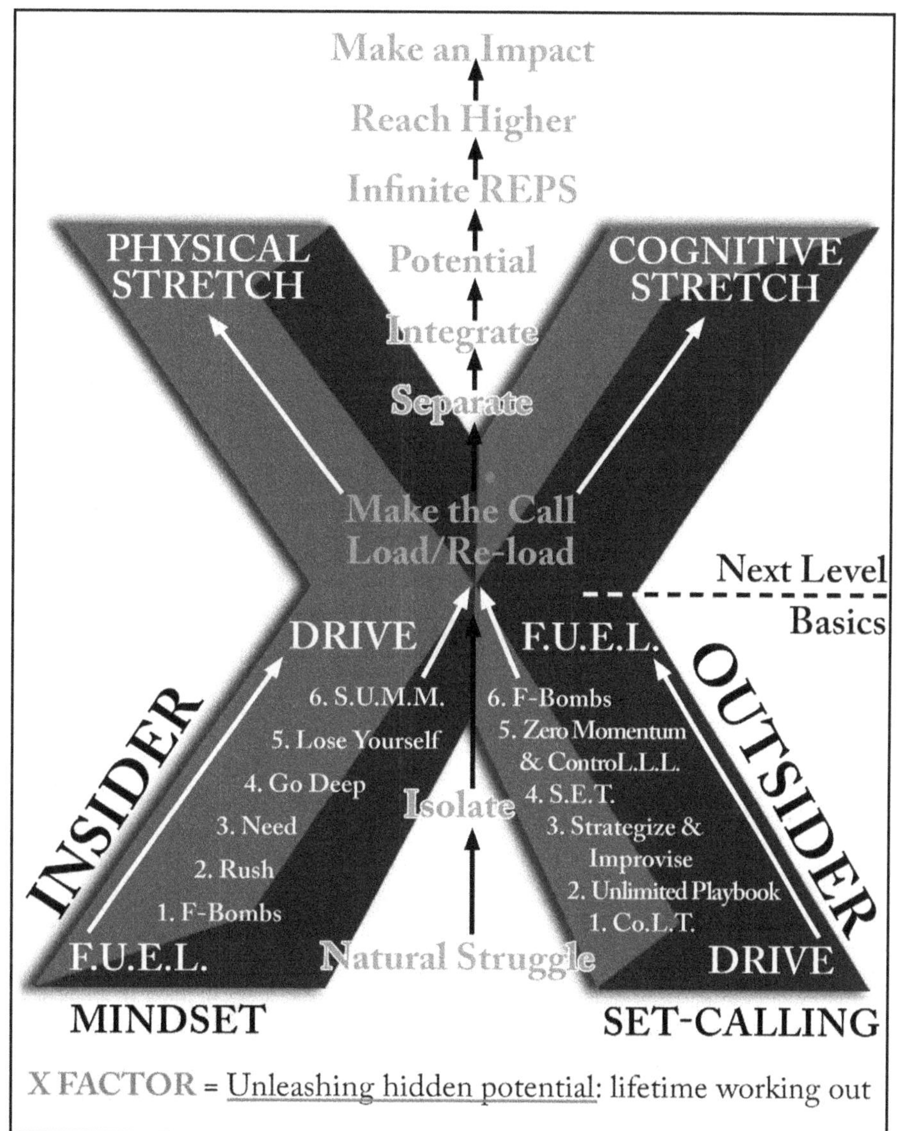

"Ora è il tempo di costruire un'enorme forza."

Now is the time to build enormous strength

Editorial #4

I am an expert on excuses because I have heard everyone ever invented. July, 2011, was a banner month for excuses – from my team and from those who want to know what's the best workout program to lose fat overnight and build muscle at warp-speed.

The best workout program has 3 elements:

- It's the one you don't miss,
- It's the one that you actually do, and
- It's the one that you spill your guts doing.

The first secret is "just show up." The second secret is work like a farm animal after you show up. The actual workout program is irrelevant if you fail to appear. If you don't show up, there is no workout in the world that will work. And no workout will help if the workout becomes an extension of social networking.

The third secret is stop eating junk. No workout has ever been invented to counter junk food consumption. Eating and drinking garbage can't be canceled out by working out. Stop blaming the workout, the equipment, your coach, or any other target of your wrath for not losing fat. Blame your food and beverage decisions. Blame your lack of willpower. Blame your weakness. Blame yourself. Stand in the mirror and point directly to the cause.

There's another secret – stay away from enablers. An enabler is any person who develops, promotes, or rewards your weaknesses. An enabler is a co-conspirator that builds softness – an accomplice who gives your weaknesses strength. An enabler is a party to the offence of rationalizing irrationalization, the skill of justifying the avoidance of work by self-deception. Rationalizing irrationalization is expert alibi-making – high performance self-bullshitting that leads to delusion and illusion.

The excuses I've heard this month are on the professional level. There is a progression of excuse-making. It starts with amateur excuses…inexperienced, rookie excuse-making. With practice, excuse-making reaches the next-level – professional. The big leagues. Expert excuse-making. Chronic excuses that block whatever it is you're trying to accomplish. The problem with professional excuse-making is curing it. The deeper the bullshit, the harder it is to purge it. The solution is an excuse-making detox. A cleansing of bullshit. Purge it before it really piles up.

Lastly, check the calendar. As each day passes, you are getting older. Old is not a number. Old is measured by inactivity. Old is the stoppage of playing. Old is living vicariously through others. Old is walking slower, talking slower, thinking slower…doing slower. Being slower. Old is standing still. Old is a state of mind that raises the white flag – surrender the fight – giving up at any age. Scolding others for what you got scolded for when you were young.

Old is retiring from the human race, retiring from planet Earth. Old is a lower pulse. Old is shutting down the hormones – letting your adrenaline gland rust.

Old is when your pension matters more than your passion. Old is when you let your dreams die – dream-slaughter, dreamicide, or simply dream-death by natural causes.

Every workout you miss, every excuse you make, is another giant step to getting old while your birth certificate says you're young.

Case Study #8: Workout Debt

I have never called myself a personal trainer. I have never asked a human being to be a client. My business card says "Football Coach" & "Strength Coach." I only coach two groups of people in the gym – football players and those who ask to be trained. The reason is the *'rule of voluntariness'* – people I coach must attend the gym free from external inducement. No external inducement to appear at the gym, no external inducement to stay in the gym. The only force that counts is internal inducement – the client's conscience has to force him/her to show up. Free to attend and free to leave at any time. No one is detained against their will. 100% voluntariness. Otherwise, it's impossible for a physical and mental makeover to happen. Free will has to be exercised for transformation to happen.

In the span of 3 months in 2011, four clients repeated what hundreds of football players have tried to do – get out of workout debt. *'I have to miss two weeks of workouts because of (insert excuse). I'll do extra sets before or after to catch up."*

Coaching moment: **You can't pay off workout debt. You can't save up workouts.** Like sleep, you can't catch up on lost workouts. Unlike money, you can't save up sets and reps. Consistency is the secret. Nothing endures without consistency. A chain of workouts is the only way to transform body and mind. Daily investment is the only way to get maximum return – a continuum of sets and rep. Inconsistent workouts will never endure. Results won't last.

Part 4.1:
The Science of Working-out

The 10% Bodyfat Rule

Body-fat is an enemy. So is mind-fat. The accumulation of both is excess baggage – the only type of heavy weight that is counter-productive. There's a line of demarcation between lean and mush – 10%. The line that separates chiseled from flabby is 10% body-fat and 10% mind-fat. That's the threshold between hard and soft.

Over 10% body-fat is easy to spot. You can pick it out of any lineup because it spills out at you. Over 10% mind-fat is easy to pick out because there's a direct connection between physical and mental fat. Soft mind, soft body – and vice-versa. Cause and effect...and side-effect. You don't need special testing to determine mind-fat percentage. There are enough symptoms of over 10% mind-fat including the Big 3:

- Excuse-making
- Rationalizing irrationality
- Physical retirement

Excuse-making speeds up rationalizing irrationality, which speeds up physical retirement way before 65. The Chain of Lethargy. Over 10% mindfat will build up over 10% bodyfat – guaranteed.

The secret to body and mind fat loss is redefining pleasure:

- The truth hurts. The truth is painful. The key to reducing body-fat percentage is reducing mind-fat percentage first. Fat loss starts at the top – mindset. If the mindset doesn't change, neither will body-fat. Changing the mindset changes the mind-fat and leading to loss of body-fat.

- Change your perception about food and working out and you'll change your appearance. An iron-will mindset is the answer to getting chiseled. The psychology of the iron-will mindset is simple – ***food as fuel, workout is a basic survival need.*** Convert pain to pleasure. Focus on feeling the rush instead of rushing away from a positive lifestyle change. Focus on the rush of eating right to fuel the rush of a workout instead of focusing on the pain of not eating junk food, not drinking junk beverage, and the pain of not sitting on your ass. In other words re-define pleasure. That's the objective of the X Fitness System.

The X Fitness System builds the X-shape.

The **X-shaped** physique is the combination of two **V-shapes**:

- V-shaped upper body, and
- inverted V-shape – powerful legs.

The X-shape is the whole package, far superior to the Y-shape (V-torso on stick legs) or the arrow-shape (love-handles on stick legs).

∞

Editorial #5

X Fitness is a social networking monster. Enormous popularity. Facebook presence.

X Fitness maxed out at 5,000 "friends" in 2 months. Then it spilled over to 3 more sites. And there's a waiting list with hundreds of "friends" waiting to be confirmed.

Hundreds press "like" to motivational posts. Hundreds more send rave reviews to commend X Fitness for inspiring them.

On July 27, 2011, X Fitness posted the following fact:

"2,282 reps ....part of a 4-day workout program guaranteed to lean you out without compromising strength. Fat loss with strength gain. – from the X Fitness training manual"

No *"likes."* No rave reviews. No '*thank you for being an inspiration.*' Why? The truth is painful. The truth hurts. Reality is not inspiring. 2,282 reps spread over 4 days is not pleasurable to most people. The truth is that 2,282 reps over 4 days works. But that message doesn't create an image of instant gratification. That's why so many mental 'dislikes' were pressed.

But, 2,282 reps over 4 days was a massive pump – physically, intellectually, emotionally, spiritually. I needed to do it. Basic survival need. Mindset – I need it and I love it. 2,282 reps didn't pop up out of nowhere. It's part of a continuum, a seamless path of workouts, all structured using **Set-Calling©** decisions.

The X Factor System

The **X Factor System** is a road map to the **X-shape**. The system is a blueprint to naturally building armour and maxing out every fiber you have. And, the system is a one-page summary of the **X Fitness System** – a step-by-step guide to teaching and learning the system.

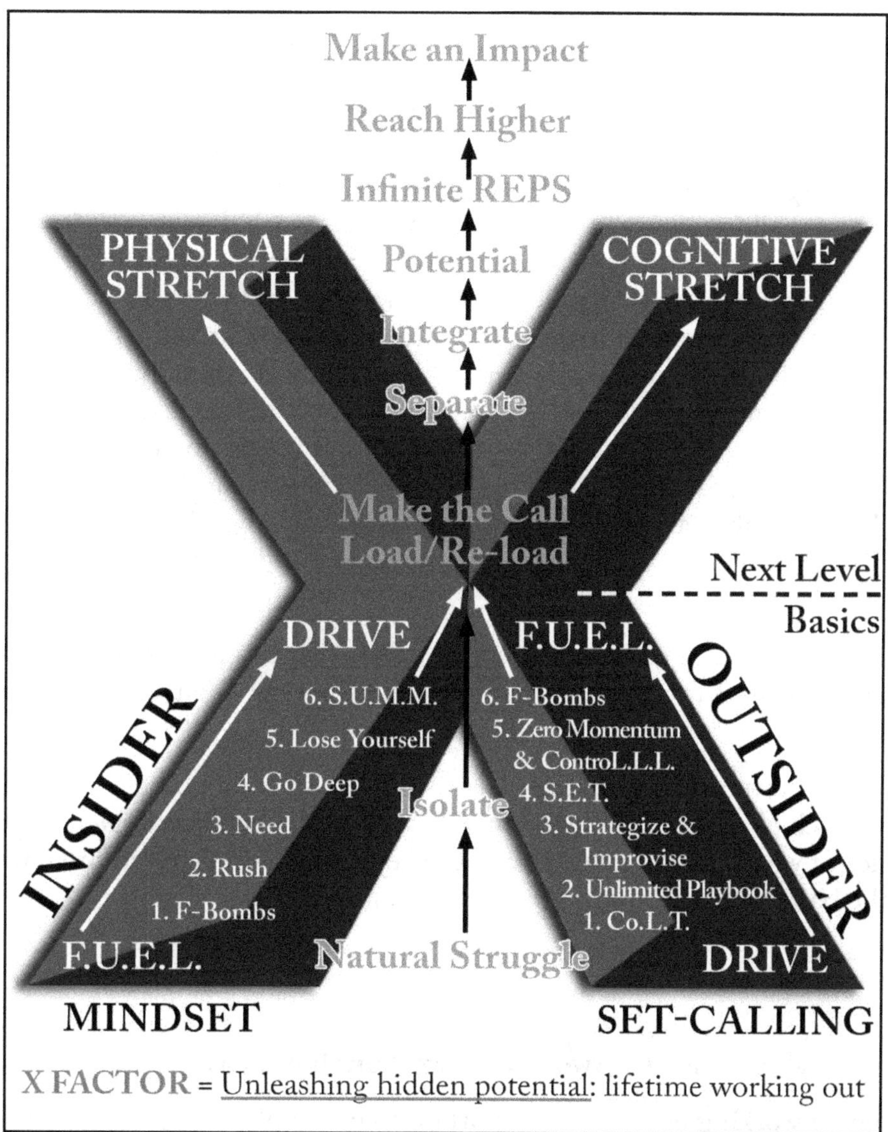

The physiology, psychology, and philosophy of the **X Fitness System** is summarized and illustrated in the **X Factor Chart**, a model based on a simple theory – there are ***infinite levels*** of performance. Unlimited levels of mental and physical performance. Contrary to popular myth, strength training is not neatly divided into 3 clear categories of beginner, intermediate, advanced. These 3 groups are *general* performance levels but they are not the total number of levels. There are *countless next levels.*

Every level of the **X** Factor has two phases – basics and stretch. The **basics** phase is characterized by and features minimal change – same exercises, same sequence but changing weight, sets, reps, and rest. The **basics** of every level form a neural pathway for each level that you progress to

– second-nature habitual movements that remove fear of the bar. The basics build the foundation for each higher training level. The basics are needed for ***stability***. You cannot stretch yourself until you have mastered the level you are at. Master the basics, then stretch. This rule applies at every level you reach. No exceptions.

The basics at every level – rookie or expert – is premised on one simple rule - Don't ignore simplicity. Don't complicate. Complexities are often the product of ego and narcissism.Working out does not need the intrigue and mystery of quantum physics. Find something heavy and lift it.

The **stretch** phase is the extreme ***shock-the-body*** stage, forcing the body to adapt to greater stress by exploding with stronger muscles and less fat. A personal ***Culture Shock***. The stretch phase is a type of ***guerilla ontology***[2], a radical transformation of mind and body, the kind every human craves and strives for. We are all wired to move toward constant growth. Every human has the seeds of potential hidden inside, waiting to be cultivated in order to surface. Our physical and mental development is not an option, it's a demand...a demand put on us by nature. Meeting that demand moves us toward the elusive state of inner peace through alignment and balance. Failing to meet that demand, by ignoring the inner need to grow physically and mentally, builds an unpleasant condition – ***cognitive dissonance***[3], defined as mental conflict... the stress of not doing what you're meant to do, capable of doing, and should be doing. Cognitive dissonance is agony... the inner turmoil of underachieving, of not reaching full potential, of wasting the talents and gifts you've been blessed with. The only way to lift the crushing weight of cognitive dissonance is by resolving the inner conflict through change – changing your mindset and changing what you do. Lifting weights lifts the weight.

You can't bypass the basics at any level. There's a ladder that has to be climbed. Every step has to be taken. The basics must become automatic – second-nature. Then, the stretch phase stretches limits and breaks them by changing the workout program.

The sequence never reverses. The stretch phasc is not the starting point – it cannot precede the basics. The stretch phase follows the basics, at every level. The ***Stretch Phase*** is grueling. It's a demanding series of workout programs. Here's the key – high-level stretch programs are goals to set sights on. The basics are ***included*** in the stretch program.

∞

Mindset and Set-Calling© are the two keys to workout longevity.

The psychology of working out is more important than the physiology of working out because without the right mindset, the physical part won't happen. The attitude toward working out and the decisions made during every single workout determine how strong or how lean you get, or... how soft and smooth you get. Mind-set toward work is the secret. Working out is therapeutic. It's a life-altering experience. But, working out is hard... ***work***. The reason why it's called ***working*** out is because of the central activity – ***work***. The harder you work, the greater the reward. The less you work, the greater the pain – the pain of frustration and failure. Work ethic affects the decisions made during a workout about ***selection*** – exercise selection, weight selection, set selection, rep selection. Work ethic is connected to ***making the call*** about how much weight to put on

2 A concept introduced by Robert Anton Wilson. Refer to bibliography.

3 A concept introduced by the esteemed researcher, Leon Festinger. Refer to bibliography.

the bar, how many sets, how many reps, and what exercise to do. Working out consistently, for a lifetime is brutally hard but it's worth every painstaking rep. The problem is the elusive search for motivation and consistency. Only two factors determine how long and how strong your workout career will be: **mind-set and Set-Calling©**. These two factors – what you focus on and the calls you make during your workout, are the secret to lifetime working out.

∞

Natural struggle is the secret to natural strength.

Avoiding the natural struggle avoids realizing full potential. The willingness or unwillingness to endure it determines the shape you'll get. Natural struggle means the inherent steps needed to climb the ladder to full potential. The natural struggle is the path of greatest resistance that must be followed to reach your fitness destination. The unnatural struggle is the path of least resistance… the path that will get you nowhere. The struggle between earned and unearned has always and will always be the fight that determines how far you go.

90-10 rule: The natural struggle eats up 90% of the population. 10% make it, 90% get cut. Those are the stats. 90-10 applies to everything I've worked in…everything I've coached or taught. Every year tens of thousands apply for police jobs – 90% get cut, 10% make it. Every year, tens of thousands play high school football – 10% move on, 90% don't. Every year, thousands of manuscripts are started in writers' minds or on paper – 90% never get finished, only 10% see the finish line. Every year, tens of thousands try working out – 10% make it a career, 90% quit. I call it, **Performance Darwinism** – the professional natural selection process. Survival of the fittest - 10% are strong enough, 90% have to try again.

The cause of the 90-10 rule is the rigors of the natural struggle. The attacks, the knock-downs, the frustrations, disappointments… the sweat, tears, and the blood. The natural struggle is relentless, ruthless, merciless, and does not give a shit about feelings. The natural struggle has only one objective – to make you tough enough. The natural struggle has a single-minded purpose – to build your will so that free-will will get exercised the right way. No one can break its burning focus. It's impossible to make the natural struggle lighten up because if it did, you would never get to where you're supposed to go.

The natural struggle can be hell but there are no short cuts. There are only escapes. Two escapes to be exact. One escape from the hell of the struggle is simply to get out of the game. Quit. Drop out of the race. Give in. Move to the sidelines, or the stands, or the couch. Pack it in and watch others live their lives. The hell of the natural struggle calls you but it doesn't force you to stay. It gives you a choice. The struggle will let any one walk away. You don't even have to tap out. Just walk away.

The second escape is fight through hell. Stay in the game. Stay on course. Keep lifting. The problem is fighting through the hell of any struggle doesn't just happen. **The only solution is iron-will mindset** – a fearless, disciplined, committed passion…a soul on fire. Ordinary motivation isn't enough – it'll only take you so far until the pressure mounts. You need to go deeper to break through the overwhelming obstacles and adversities of the natural struggle. A burning drive is the only way to survive what the natural struggle throws at you. It's impossible to beat the odds with a weak-will. Soft minds break easily.

There is one temptation that perpetuates the greatest myth in the world of fitness and sports– that the natural struggle can be circumvented. Steroids, performance-enhancing drugs, fat-burners, stimulants... the biggest contradiction in society – a sports and fitness world that tries to project clean living and hard work is steeped in bullshit. Unnatural muscle heralded by proponents of natural means. The unhealthiest lifestyles promoted by a health and fitness industry hell-bent on selling fantasy. If steroids and all performance-enhancing drugs suddenly disappeared from planet Earth, appearances would change. Sports would not look the same. Fitness would not look the same. Reality would set it. If every sport, especially football, forced every athlete to take polygraph tests and drug tests, the nature of competition would change dramatically. If sports officials were serious about concussions, they would wage a serious war against steroid abusers and PED abusers. Leveling the playing field by chasing drug abusers should be the number-one priority for sports administrators if they truly want to protect athletes from brain injury and delusion. Steroids are not the only cause of head injuries but ignoring unnaturally stronger, bigger bodies as being a leading factor in the cause is the height of ignorance, foolishness, and neglect.

In addition to the obvious danger of your kids playing violent sports on drug-induced tilted playing fields, steroids and PEDs are a form of slow suicide. The last sudden death I investigated during my detective career is the best evidence – a freakishly strong bodybuilder died at an unnaturally young age because of internal organs that had aged faster than his body. His autopsy photos should be attached to Surgeon-General warnings on steroid packaging.

But, until steroids and PEDs vanish from the Earth, the sports and fitness industries will make the gullible believe in make-believe. And it will continue to work because bullshit really does baffle brains. Syringes and vials will continue being the replacement for the struggle for as long as they are available because hard work, true sustained physical exertion, strikes fear.

The reason why 90% quit working out is the fear of the anticipated pain associated with the natural struggle. The thought of traveling the path of greatest resistance is unappealing and unattractive. It scares and derails good intentions. Fear is fuel for temptations... the temptation is to take short cuts, the temptation for instant gratification, the temptation to avoid the frustration of impatience, and the temptation to avoid the discomfort of manual labour. Giving in to temptations of steroids and PEDs exacts a costly price financially, physically, and mentally.

First, steroids will bankrupt you and land you in jail. Secondly, they're a ticket to the morgue. Thirdly, they're artificial detours that circumvent the lessons learned by the natural struggle. Trying to take a short cut that isn't there is the equivalent of driving off the road at a high-speed. Crash. The natural struggle tests every fiber – mind and body. Steroids avert those tests, building artificial strength, physically and mentally. Steroid strength is not real. It's an illusion. The secret to avoiding a crash – change the focus. Change the focus away from the fear of the natural struggle and move the focus towards it. Head-on. Stand up to it. Don't move off the track. The secret is to need the natural struggle and demand it. Avoiding it is self-destructive. **Workout longevity is the result of beating Athletic Darwinism**. Staying in the workout game is a victory in the natural selection process. ***Survival of the strongest and fittest.*** If you pass, you move to the next level. If you fail, you get to try again.

∞

Isolation is the heaviest weight to handle.

The unwillingness and incapacity to work out in isolation severely deters the workout careers of those who constantly need some form of social interaction. We are all connected. We can't do it alone. We can't make it happen isolated from the rest of the planet...we need a team to get the best out of ourselves. But, to get to the next level, we have to work in isolation at some point – ***isolation from an audience and isolation from a team.***

Weak-will will weaken the desire to sacrifice social networking for iron set-working. Social life is the top reason for failing to appear at workouts. Absenteeism by socialism. No audience, no conscience, no patience, no experience – the Chain of Isolation. The solution is team training.

Team training is the most powerful force especially for rookies who have underdeveloped work ethic and commitment. Nothing works better for a rookie than working out with a coach and a team. Nothing comes close. But, working out alone is inevitable and necessary for two reasons. First, team training is not permanent and not always practicable. Secondly, working out alone teaches you how to ***flip the switch*** alone without any help, a necessity to develop the full power of the beast and to develop the mechanism to call out the beast. Dependence must lead to independence to move up on the strength maturity ladder.

Isolation is a temporary disconnection through separation...a separation from real or artificial social network. Isolation is painful. Isolated training is the enemy – the toughest opponent you will ever face in the gym – and the reason why 90% quit working out. How strong and muscular you get depends on how you handle the pain of working out in isolation. Beat isolation and you will dramatically improve your strength and physique. If you don't, your workouts will suffer badly – you'll never come close to reaching your full potential.

∞

Workouts are a series of decisions.

They form a chain of calls that are made about what to lift, how to lift it, when to lift, and how often. Make the right call. Designing a workout is a product of strategic decision-making that evaluates the past and present in order to predict the future. You need to know what you did in order to figure out what to do next. Some workout decisions are pre-planned ***before*** the workout but others are rapid-fire decisions that must be made ***during*** the workout. Explosive, next-level workouts depend on ***making the right call*** during a workout... in-progress structured decision-making, not randomly winging it. The formula for making the right call during a workout is found in the **Set-Calling©** model. **Set-Calling©** is a science. It's not learned overnight – skills don't just happen. First you need a coach, then you need research to know yourself. Every workout is an experiment... research – a personal case study. Study each one carefully and you will unlock the secret to making the right calls.

∞

We all have the inner beast waiting to get called out.

The inner beast is a high-power drive to reach full potential. The inner beast is capable of enormous feats of strength. The inner beast is a beast of burden work ethic that's willing and capable of overcoming the biggest odds; of doing more than we can imagine; of achieving far beyond our current expectation. The inner beast won't remain silent. It makes noise... louder and louder until it gets released. Keeping the inner beast caged up is a recipe for disaster – intense inner turmoil. The solution is simple – **call out the beast**.

∞

There is overwhelming evidence that individual potential is limitless.

We will never reach full potential while we're still alive. The goal is to keep reaching – reaching potential is a work-in-progress. There's one problem, one heavy obstacle – belief. Poor conditioning. Negative conditioning – believing that success is reserved for others. Believing that we have limited potential. Believing that potential works within a caste system, believing that we have second-class potential, or third-class... or lower. Weak mental conditioning is the product of a lifetime of myths, limitations, and restrictions hammered into our heads by the forces of conventional-thinking conformists.

Editorial #6

I have interviewed thousands of students, athletes, and adults who want advice about shaping their future. I always ask, *"What's your goal in life?"* The most popular answer in first place all by itself is, *"I want to make a difference. I want to help people."* The connection between making a difference and other people is the strongest bond that drives all of our inner beasts. Every human has the capacity to make an impact. The difference is those who listen and those who don't… those who act and those who won't. A thunderous impact on self and then on others… the choice is ours. We are free to underachieve or overachieve. We are free to limit ourselves or unlock ourselves. We are free to load or unload. We are free to make whatever choices we want. We can choose to get in the game or watch. We can choose to fight through whatever struggle is needed to reach higher or avoid it and stay put.

Yesterday, I posted yet another motivational stat from **"the X Fitness training manual**" on all my social networking sites. Here's one response I received: *"What do you suggest for a 310-pound couch potato who sits behind a desk all day?"* I receive this type of message repeatedly. Consistent pleas to please help cure the side-effects of hidden potential. We all hide our full potential to some degree. To some extent, we all bury some potential or ignore it or release it slower than we'd like. We all share the same challenge. We can start by making a small impact, then another, and another until all them become an explosion. One by one, we can impact ourselves and this world – building potential in self and then in others. It's hard work but nothing is more rewarding.

If you don't work out, start this minute. If you do, make a performance demand – insist to yourself that you will reach higher and then put up ladders for others. Making an impact is a matter of fitness – the exercise of free will.

Extraordinary drive is needed to drive you to the gym and drive you in the gym.

The actual workout program is secondary because the mind will give out long before the body. The best workout program in the world is useless if you don't have the drive to endure the endless repetition of re-construction – tearing down and re-building. The cycle of emptying the tank and re-filling over and over again is draining, mentally and physically.

Workouts are investments into your body, mind, heart, and soul. Unlike financial investments, workouts don't pay compound interest. You can't workout once and hope to get longterm returns on just that one workout. You cannot save up sets and reps that you invest in a workout. You can't conserve energy. You cannot conserve strength. The effects of one workout don't last forever. They don't last years or months or weeks or even days. It's impossible to preserve what you build. There is no long-term return on a single workout investment – no annuities, no royalties. Strength and fitness returns need daily investments.

Imagine razing a building every day and then rising it back up. Raze and rise, over and over. Workouts wreck, post-workouts fix. Working out is a demolition crew. Post-workout is the re-construction team. But, unlike structures, humans get stronger every time they're re-built. With buildings, wrecking and re-construction are two separate concepts. Not so with the human body – wrecking and fixing work together to build continuously stronger armour. Human demolition and human re-construction are connected, forming a team, a unified force... a chain of strength-building. The worse you wreck, the stronger you get. Here's the challenge – the pressure of repeating this process day in, day out is overwhelming.

Pressure makes you or breaks you. To make it, you have to fuel the mental drive. Fueling the mental drive fuels the physical drive. It takes intense, sustained determination and the highest tolerance for discomfort to empty the tank day after day. You have to do deep-sea exploration inside your heart and soul and guts to find every fiber of strength to drain the battery on a daily basis. Because emptying the tank tears down the body. Recovery – the ultimate change agent – builds a new and improved version, depending on how close the needle gets to "E." The size of the tank is infinite. It grows – if the body believes it's necessary. The closer you get to an empty tank, the bigger the tank gets. A shocked body compensates. It gets ready for bigger battles. More room for fuel.

After the demolition crew empties the tank and drains the battery, the post-workout re-construction team has to fuel and fix for the next workout with proper food and sleep. Workouts are wasted if the re-construction fails because of sub-standard building materials. Not even world-class athletes can abuse, alcohol, and substances. Getting wasted wastes workouts. Re-construction takes iron-will. The secret is to proper nutrition is a special mindset – **FOOD AS FUEL.** Viewing food as fuel for your next workout is the starting point for fat loss and replacing mush with muscle. Eat right, sleep right or it doesn't matter what workout program you follow. Using your gut as a human garburator and not sleeping enough not only keeps the tank empty, it rots the tank.

The 90-10 rule applies here – 90% will break under the pressure of re-construction – fueling and recovering properly – and eventually quit. The pleasure of beer and junk food is too tempting. **The secret to success is waste management** – manage the waste that goes into the body and mind, and reduce the wasted workout opportunities.

Workout deprivation leads to workout retirement which leads to the heaviest weight of all – regret. Workout deprivation starts the mad scramble to make up for lost time. You can't make up for workout deprivation. You can't pay off workout debt. Once you sink into workout debt, you don't start where you left off... you start deep in the red, far below zero.

F-bombs are the key to iron-will mind-set.

The philosophy I've shared with tens of thousands of football players and college law enforcement students is: **soft mind, hard landing**. A weak mind will get you a crash landing, flat on your ass on the field or in real-life.

During two decades of teaching and coordinating college law enforcement programs, I witnessed countless **REPS** (**Re**-cycled **E**xcuses **P**romoting **S**ympathy) from applicants after failing to pass the police selection process: physical testing, intellectual testing, psychological testing, interviews, background checks. *"I got screwed." "The interview was unfair." "The scoring was…"* Every excuse imaginable to evoke sympathy to soften the crash landing of reality. The search for sympathy connects to another set of **REPS** (**R**ecruiting **E**nablers **P**romotes **S**oftness). Enablers are accomplices who reward soft minds by adding energy to imagined conspiracy theories. Enablers fuel weak-will by confirming delusions. Enablers make the soft softer.

The same applies to football. During forty seasons of coaching, I've heard all rookie REPS for losing imaginable – refs, teammates, field conditions, uniforms… anything but the truth.

Coaching moment: *After you get knocked on your ass, immediately send yourself one simple two-word message –* **my fault.** *Then, say it out loud. Two announcements of the truth – private, then public – are the first steps to changing a mush mind-set. Spare yourself and everyone around you the bullshit of blame. Excuse-making is a complete waste of time…valuable time that should be invested in changing the real culprit – weakness. If you fail to get what you want, you weren't ready. Train harder.*

My mental makeover formula is the F-bomb:

Focus + Feedback = Fuel. **What you focus on grows. Change the focus, change the outcome.**

My biggest challenge as a coach and college teacher has been training student-athletes to focus. It's the single-most draining part of the job. **Full concentration** is the key to maximizing any experience. **Intense focus** on what you're doing keeps you doing it longer until you reach the big leagues… expert-level. But focus takes work. It's painful. Broken focus guarantees losing. Distractions guarantee derailment. Getting side-tracked is easy. People look for, and are easily influenced by anything that takes their eyes off the ball. When any job gets to tough, distractions not only are temptation, they become a welcomed relief.

I have never actually told any athlete or student to "focus." I have never used the word 'focus' during a workout, a practice, or a game. Telling someone to 'focus' is not enough. It's a waste of breath to actually say "*focus on the workout*" or "*focus on this drill*" because focus is an outcome. It doesn't tell them how to do it, it only alerts them to the intended result. Focus is a skill that has to be taught and learned. It doesn't just happen. The attention span of rookies I coach in the gym, on the field, or in the classroom is shockingly low. One of my biggest challenges is to expand the attention span. It's impossible to retain anything physically or mentally without that capacity for a long attention span. Muscle memory (physically and mentally) is directly proportionate to attention span. How long you can focus determines how strong you get – body, mind, and soul.

The depth of your attention span is the difference between eliminating waste from your workouts and wasting your time. Reps are not created equal. There are ordinary reps and extraordinary reps. Ordinary reps are low-impact reps. Extraordinary reps are high-impact reps. How strong you get depends on how long you can lose yourself during a workout and how much a workout can make you lose your old self. How do you lose yourself? High-impact reps: reps that lead to an *eXplos*ive experience, a unique type of rush that I call **S.U.M.M.** – **S**ubjectively **U**nique **M**eaningfulness = **M**emorable.

The secret to workout longevity is building a chain of S.U.M.M. experiences that separate themselves from all the rest of what you do. When they are so different, so original, so powerful, your workout becomes an *eXplos*ion. A magnet that brings you back for more. Back to the same place and the same new self – the one who ignited the explosion. That's how you fuel the drive to keep working out – how you build the beast. Without fueling the drive, the flame goes out.

High-impact reps transform mind and body by demanding and absorbing a full tank of energy. No energy conservation, just energy depletion. I'm not referring to a type of exhaustion that induces vomiting, shaking, feinting, seizure, or any other unnatural, uncontrolled, or involuntary bodily function or response. If any of those happen, go to the hospital and get checked out physically and mentally. An empty tank is the explosive experience, the combination of natural stimulant and natural cleanse – a purging of built-up pollution, waste, and junk piled up by real-life combined with high-octane fuel that rejuvenates, re-energizes, re-builds, and restores. The gym is not the only place where the explosive experience can be achieved. It happens any time you give 100% physically or intellectually or emotionally or spiritually to an assignment. Professionally or personally. The explosive experience heals an ailing mind, body, and soul because it brings to life **meaning**.

Meaning is the greatest power that lights a soul on fire. Meaning is soul nourishment that spread to body and mind. Replenishing a tired, aching soul replenishes a tired, aching body and mind. "Meaning" is the anabolic agent of all growth – physical, intellectual, emotional, and spiritual. Injecting meaning is the quickest, safest, most legal way to build muscle fiber, mind fiber, and soul fiber.[4]

There's a long road to going deep. It's impossible to lengthen attention span overnight from short-distance to long-distance. Attention span is expanded one impact rep at a time. Start at the surface and starting moving deeper one rep at a time…until you go as deep as your mind lets you.

Instant feedback is a powerful motivator. The most motivating jobs in the world are those that give you an immediate score. Coaching football is a great example. Call a play, watch it unfold, and get instant feedback – explosive play or busted-up play. And there's a giant scoreboard that flashes the score (unless you coach football in Canada where the 90-10 rule applies – 90% of Canadian football fields have no scoreboard). The worst jobs are those where you have no idea what the score is, no idea if you making the great calls or stupid calls, no feedback whatsoever.

The gym is one strategy for the mental makeover. **Iron will build iron-will.** Working out is one of those activities that gives you immediate feedback – instant messaging about failure to reach failure or successfully reaching failure. Or, passing the 20-rep finish line for 225-lb bench press and squats.

Focus and feedback are the primary ingredients for workout fuel, the secret to the **mindset makeover…** the transformation of weak-will to iron-will. The mental makeover doesn't just happen and it doesn't happen overnight. The starting point is the paradigm shift…re-defining pain and pleasure.

---

4 Tribute to a masterpiece, *Man's Search For Meaning* (1946) by Dr. Viktor Frankl. One of the most influential books of the 20th century. The book is divided into 2 parts. Part 1 decribes Dr. Frankl's experience as a Holocaust survivor. Part 2 explains his theory of Logotherapy that focuses on the will to meaning. Meaning is the drive that keep human's going. The absence of meaning is a hell on Earth.

Changing the focus from the **pain of work to the thrill of the rush** is the secret to repetition that leads to career longevity. Changing the mindset from pain to pleasure makes you want to do it again – and again. More and more – can't get enough. This change of focus **FLIPS THE SWITCH.** Switch 'on' calls out the beast. Switch 'off' turns the beast against yourself. It's impossible to enjoy a long workout career without changing the focus from pain to pleasure. It can't be done. The anticipation of the rush and experiencing the actual effects of the rush are the keys to not quitting.

∞

Rush: The vaccine for boredom and anxiety.

The key to reaching peak performance is winning the struggle between boredom and anxiety[5] – the never-ending inner conflict between the monotony of unchallenging routine and the terror of being under-skilled for a challenge. Left unchecked, both anxiety and boredom has the same side-effect – quitting. The rush is the cure for both boredom and anxiety. H-bombs – hormone blasts. But the switch is flipped only in one place – striking the balance between anxiety and boredom. Finding the line of demarcation that separates underachieving from overwhelming – from inexperienced to overqualified.

Every workout must strike this balance to achieve maximum benefits. Every set must has the same objective – find the line that flips the switch.

∞

Need it – Demand it: The Power of the Performance Demand.

Need is the difference between half-assed mediocrity and extraordinary results. Need is the difference between those who beat the odds and those who let the odds beat them. Need is the difference between those who take working out seriously – take ***anything*** seriously - and those who don't give a shit. Need is the difference between those who endure and those who give up the minute things get tough. Need is the difference between the strong and the weak. Need is the difference between those who make it happen and those who hate, envy, despise, resent, complain about, and hold in contempt those who do make it happen.

I have been asked thousands of times about how to get motivated to workout. My answer is ***find a need.*** Find something that will flip the switch. Find a reason to get passionate. If you can't find one, build it…build a need to work out. If you still can't, you're not trying or you're lying to yourself. Find a coach – a ***mentor*** - who will teach you how to find a need and how to keep building it.

At first, my answer is not what they're looking for. They prefer to hear bullshit about how to drag their ass to a gym – romantic, pie-in-the-sky, tear-jerking fairy tales about how to change apathy and lethargy overnight. The reason is that building a compelling need takes effort, intensity, and an outpouring of locked up desire and passion. In other words, it takes work – sustained work to build a powerful need.

5 The work of Dr. Mihaly Csikszentmihalyi (1990) *Flow: The Psychology of Optimal Experience.* New York: Harper and Row. ISBN 0-06-092043-2 , has made a deep impact on my teaching/coaching ideology. I included and referenced his theory of a state of "flow" in literature reviews for both my M.Ed. and partial PhD dissertation. Dr. Csikszentmihalyi's seminal research concluded that both anxiety and boredom have the same negative effect – they block peak performance. Reaching the balance achieves optimal experience. But finding the elusive balance is easier said than done. The X Fitness System strives to find a concrete blueprint by applying some of the "flow" principles.

Case Study #9: Brutally Honest Truth

One of the most bizarre questions I have ever been asked was at a college recruiting night (in April). A grown man in his 20's, who wanted to be a cop, grabbed his gut, pulled a handful of flab, and asked me, *"I let myself go. How can I get rid of this before September?"*

Coaching moment: *"You won't because you don't need to. You don't need to be a cop. You like the idea of it but you don't desperately need it. If you did really need to be a cop, you wouldn't have let yourself go, you wouldn't embarrass yourself by what you just did, and you wouldn't disrespect the profession."* Silence. I honestly believe I was the first person who ever told him the truth – the brutally honest reality. I believe I was the first person not to enable his delusions.

Two years later at convocation, the same guy told me he never forgot what I told him and that my honesty changed his life. His gut was gone, made it on the honour roll, and got hired as a cop 18 months later. He still works out.

Case Study #10: Need

A perfectly healthy 20-year-old football player asked me in June, *"Like, how can I get my 225 bench better this year so I can get a scholarship? I haven't worked out for awhile you know because like I've been stressed out with school and stuff, you know, like it's been hectic like...."*

Coaching moment: *"You won't ever get your 225 bench or squats up to scholarship level until you need it. You don't give a shit about yourself or the sport. When you decide you need it, you'll respect yourself and respect the game."* He played on my team for 2 years. He worked out religiously. His personal bests upon graduation were 16 reps at 225 bench press and 22 reps at 225 squats. He earned a partial scholarship, went to university, had a successful career, and graduated with honours. He is currently in the selection process for police hiring after failing to get hired twice before. Recently, he told me that my brutal honesty changed his life. He no longer makes excuses, no longer cracks under the disappointment of setbacks, and is committed to constantly improve until he gets hired.

My coaching speeches and college lectures always include a warning: *"If you fail to get what you want, you didn't need what you failed to get."* I send that same message over and over. I never soften the message because I would be a liar if I told them they could get what they want by being lazy, lethargic, apathetic sluggards.[6]

Need is the most powerful motivator.

Wanting isn't enough. Wishing isn't enough. Positive thinking isn't enough. "Need" flips the switch, triggering a force of nature called the **performance demand**, a no-choice, no-alternative, no-escape assignment that becomes a mission. A passion. A performance demand is a Zero Tolerance policy that stems from a Zero Tolerance ideology. Zero Tolerance means ineptitude, incompetence, half-assed mediocrity. **Personal and team performance is direct evidence of what you do and don't tolerate.** Performance is the universal language that communicates your personal competence and team's competence. Success and failure is directly connected to how much apathy and lethargy you tolerate...or don't. I have repeatedly told players and students: *"You are a walking billboard of your performance and tolerance level."* Appearance matters to recruiters in both football and law enforcement. Performance and tolerance/intolerance levels are connected by an inverse relationship. Performance skyrockets as intolerance for apathy, lethargy, and ineptitude plummets. Conversely, your performance sinks into an abyss if your tolerance for laziness grows, guaranteeing a role of sub-par, back-of-the-pack weight for a team to carry. Same applies to leadership of any kind. Leadership is measured by levels of tolerance, what is promoted and what is prohibited. Performance demands on self and team are a by-product and expression of Zero Tolerance for failure outside the gym and for the discomfort of failure in the gym. **The pain of losing hurts more than the pain invested in winning.** Change the focus, change the outcome.

---

6 A tribute to two masterpieces: (i) *Light my Fire* by Jim Morrison and the Doors; and (ii) *Book of Proverbs*, where Solomon uses '*sluggard*' 14 times to describe and scold the chronically lazy.

Making a performance demand on self is the highest level of self-discipline. It's an inner drive that will not accept any bad news, frustrations, obstacles, adversity, or any barrier as an excuse to give up. Making a performance demand on a team is the highest level of leadership and the single-most important and challenging coaching skill. The ability to make performance demands separates great leaders from incompetent leaders. It separates winning coaches from losing coaches, successful business owners from broke business owners, memorable teachers from forgettable teachers, true mentors from ordinary instructors. The gift of making performance demands will separate you from the rest.

There's much more to coaching and mentoring than simply teaching someone how to hold a bar, how to lift it, how many times to do it, what to eat, and what not to eat. The true measure of a coach/mentor is whether s/he can teach someone else how to make self-performance demands – how to call out their own inner beast. Coaching impact is measured by the **stretch distance** – how far the coach can stretch another person's potential.

It's impossible to make performance demands on someone else if you can't make your own. **You can't demand from others what you don't demand of self.** There's a two stage performance demand-making process. First you have to conquer the inner sluggard by making self-performance demands, on demand. Afterward, share the secret – teach teams of people how to do the same. Vice-versa doesn't work. Performance demands by those unwilling or incapable of making their own, have no weight.

The difference between a performance demand and a request is the presence or absence of choice. A request allows a decision – two choices. Make it happen or don't. A request lets free will get exercised. Performance demands give only one choice – make it happen. The second alternative is not available. No decision, no escape. What's the secret to learning how to make performance demands? Turn ordinary need to basic survival need. The performance demand naturally follows. It becomes automatic.

Needs are not created equal. The most potent needs are survival needs – the basics needed to stay alive… food, water, shelter to name a few. The secret is **add to that list.** Whatever you add becomes a basic survival need. It becomes deeply ingrained in your lifestyle. You won't live without it. Having it is not an option. I've worked out uninterrupted for 42 years because I've made working out a basic survival need. My teams have won championships because they made working out a basic survival need. That's been the secret to the winning transformation, changing losing cultures to winning cultures. I've done the same with every part of my professional and personal life. It worked in business, with a 24-hour gym that I started, a traditional risky business that became more treacherous when the city started crumbling economically a year later. It worked with writing. I managed to achieve a 100% publishing rate in the most challenging publishing field – law enforcement academic textbooks, literature that wasn't popular with publishers and with readers. It worked in getting hired and surviving 15 years in frontline policing. It worked in college teaching, where I was given a goal to raise enrolment so I did – quadrupled it. And it worked in football, where I've been head coach of six different programs that had previously never experienced winning. Making each challenge a basic survival need guaranteed performance demands that were met – on self and on my teams.

The only way to workout consistently and reach full potential is to deepen the need. Once working out and the need to feel the rush become basic survival needs, you will never quit working out and you will never squander a workout. Not one set, not even a rep. Like an environmentalist, you will eliminate all waste. The key to building a deep need is the depth of hunger, a mind-set that the mind will resist at first but eventually adopt to. The mind loves conformity and comfort. The mind wants you to blend into the mainstream – disappear in the crowd. Live by the conventional-thinking rulebook. Throw away originality. Douse the fire inside. Put on sheepskin and follow the crowd. Assimilate instead of innovate. The secret is to separate from the rest by separating from the rest. The driving force behind performance demands is a blue-collar work ethic… the willing to get some stains – sweat, dirt, and even some blood.

How do you make working out a basic survival need? Every basic survival need has a fear-driven force. Something you're trying to avoid with all your heart and soul. Nothing changes until you need to change. And needing to change is driven by fear-avoidance – a need to avert the worst-case scenario. What you can't stand the most you will passionately avoid.

Here's how I built my list of fear-driven forces. My first one was the need, as a child, to change obesity, a nightmare that I'm driven to avoid. My fight with fat has become a life-long battle. It doesn't go away. Obesity is something I refuse to return to. But avoiding obesity doesn't just happen. It takes excruciating work, self-discipline, and top-level performance demands. Preventing obesity was first on my list, at the age of 12. Then I kept adding to the list. The same year, I added fear of football embarrassment – had to stop getting knocked on my ass physically and verbally as a little leaguer preparing to go to the next level – high school. Obese children are targets for blame by asshole coaches and asshole teammates. Changing that became a passion. Six years later, I became driven to avoid getting killed or maimed in front-line policing. The CSI-bullshit warps public perception of policing. It's not the sexy glamorous action-hero fantasy world that Hollywood portrays. The reality is you can get killed. The frontline can chew you up if you're not ready to handle it. Policing is Reality Darwinism – survival of the fittest, extinction of the weakest. Nine years later, I added to the list with the fear of my players getting killed or maimed on the playing field. Protecting other peoples' blessings is the most difficult job I've ever had. Coaching a violent sport is not for dumb-ass loiterers who live vicariously through their kids, guaranteeing a starting position for their daughter or son by sporting an ill-fitting golf shirt stitched with "Coach". Coaching football requires more life experience than playing Madden video games in your basement. The fear of someone else's pride and joy getting busted up on the playing field propelled my workouts to a level I never imagined – leading and coaching by example. Then, my colleagues and inner circle added to my list. They scared the shit out me by becoming senior citizens prematurely. I was driven to avoid premature aging. Then, my favourite number, my high school jersey number – 51 – pushed me to even higher levels when it appeared on a birthday card. That day, my workouts sky-rocketed. No one I've coached has out-lifted or out-lasted me in the gym… and it won't ever happen. Working out is the ultimate anti-aging secret. Working out consistently, throughout a lifetime, is the difference between becoming a senior citizen on your 30th birthday and staying young regardless of your date of birth – the difference between how old you are and how long you've been alive.

The common denominator for every fear-driven force that was added to my list was "iron deficiency." A daily mega-dose of iron is required. That's why I never take prolonged time off. My goal is to work out 26 out of 28 days. One day off, clouds form. Two days off brings on a storm. Can't imagine the typhoon of three days off or more. The real pain – an ***unbearable*** pain – would be not being able to work out. The real pain of deteriorating workouts followed by quitting and early retirement and immediately growing old. Make your experience ***eXplode*** and you'll never grow old. That's why I give thanks after every workout… "Thank you God Almighty for letting me do this."

Case Study #11: "Make Me Puke"

"Make me puke." One of the craziest requests I've ever been asked. A fitness competitor who I had never met in my life – a complete stranger – asked me to coach her in the gym to help prepare her for a stage competition. *"Make me puke"* was her misguided solution to her underachieving that had plagued her career. *"Make me puke"* was her ludicrous perception of my coaching ideology that she had wrongly interpreted from a friend of hers' whom I had coached. *"Make me puke"* was not her fault. She simply bought into the myth... the bullshit that getting violently ill is a sign of intensity.

Coaching moment: "I don't make people puke. I have never puked in my life. I'm not a doctor but puking is a symptom that something's wrong. A sign that something's not working right. A symptom of poor health. Puking is unnatural. There's a clear line between emptying the tank and medical exhaustion that empties the stomach. Draining the battery does not mean crossing the line to a condition where the body loses its ability to function properly. Intentionally inviting sickness is a sign of a deeper problem – conformity, easily influenced, misguided, or even worse... a need for self-abuse. Emptying the tank is a feeling of renewal and empowerment, not incapacitation."

CoLT: **Co**ach-**L**ed**T**eam is the secret to explosive workouts.

People who consistently reach the next level in fitness by training alone are rare – extremely rare. I have never coached a rookie who consistently climbed the ladder by training alone. The rare person who can do it has to be powered by a special kind of inner force that's fueled by a deep-rooted need and the ability. One that can flip the switch to make consistent self-performance demands day after painstaking day. That inner force is a soul of a lifter on fire. A red-hot, burning soul of a lifter is the ultimate coach, an inner force that builds an iron-will that will drive through any barrier. It's an inner force that just won't quit. The soul of a lifter on fire is an inner beast that gets called out by simply flipping the switch – no other people necessary. The majority of those who try to work out alone never consistently climb to the next level or end up quitting. The reason is that a soul of lifter on fire has to be built-up...developed. It doesn't just happen. Every human has the potential soul of a lifter, one that can lift something heavy and, more importantly, one that can lift another person. And therein lies the secret to exploding – souls of lifters uniting into one force of nature.

Our consistent team workouts have never failed to dramatically improve rookies and veterans. Female or male, whatever sport or job or personal goal, my team workouts have a 100% success rate for improvement. Not one person got weaker or fatter or skinner or softer. These are bold statements but they're backed up by evidence – physical evidence and witnesses. The operative word is "consistent." Team workouts have a 100% success rate when the people don't fail to appear. The worst gym crime is fail to appear. Nothing happens when you fail to appear. You have to drive yourself to get to gym. My job is to drive people *in* the gym. I won't contribute to the coddling of society by cajoling, coaxing, and otherwise pleading with people to work out, including my own players. Life is about choices. So is working out. The only way to strengthen free will is to exercise it regularly in the direction of the gym. The drive to the gym is the easy part. The drive in the gym is the hard part. If someone can't drive to the gym, they aren't ready for the drive in the gym.

The phenomenon of team workouts has to be experienced to be fully understood but the following is how it happens and what results from them:

- **How it happens** – Why do team workouts dramatically improve individual strength & conditioning?
- **Shared-misery.** One of the strongest bonding agents is surviving hell together. Shared-misery has been my best team-building exercise. It's been the fastest, most powerful way to unify a team of complete strangers. I never have and never will use pizza nights, retreats, campfires, kayaking trips, hiking, movie nights or beer bashes to build team unity. If a team wants to socialize together, it has to be voluntary. They have to want to be there. Personally, I can't stand forcing people to socialize because I can't stand being forced to socialize. It's juvenile and arrogant to assume that you know who someone wants to spend time with off the field or away from the gym. It's a form of mind-control. Brainwashing. Making people believe that they have to act, talk, behave in a certain way as dictated by the team leader, to be socially accepted through assimilation – surrendering originality for the privilege of adding to your friends count. Sing-songs, karaoke, may work for junior kindergarten and frat parties but not for high-risk violent activities where not getting killed or maimed is the top priority. What has worked for us is the cosmic force of suffering through and surviving some discomfort, a departure from the ordinary, uneventful, sedentary routine of life. Surviving hell binds a team tighter than shared DNA.
- **Separation anxiety.** Survival of the fittest is contagious. No one wants to get cut because s/he couldn't take it. Seeing your peers endure struggle builds a healthy fear of being left behind. Getting separated from a group of beasts becomes the worst nightmare. The need to survive Athletic Darwinism is a powerful motivator. Needing to be make the cut along with your peers is high octane fuel that pushes you past any beast that stands in your way.
- **Need to be part of something.** Most people fall into the trap of mundane routine. Boredom and meaninglessness become heavy weight to carry. Monotony triggers a search, a quest for more. The need grows to become part of something…something bigger than self, something with greater meaning – a higher purpose. Teams inject new meaning into individual lives by trying to collectively stretch through the pursuit of higher purpose. Sticking to a job is easier when you're part of a hungry team that's searching for the same thing you are. Being part of something is switch-stimulating – it ***flips the switch.***
- **Challenge to go big or go home**. Every human dreams big – or should. Dreams make you push past limits that imprison your soul. If your big dreams stop, you're in big trouble. Teams take on big challenges that require traveling…traveling so far outside the box until the box disappears. The challenge to go big or go home revs up the inner generator. Having to choose between the two makes you confront your fears – another switch-stimulator. To go big, you have to learn to think, play, and work outside the box. It's easier to move outside the box when you've got passengers. Team travel is better than driving alone. Moving outside the box is infectious. First you see your peers do it, then you try it. The experience becomes addictive. Life outside the box that had confined you, has a magnetic attraction. You won't go back inside the box once your mind, body, and soul leave it.
- **Fearlessness by committee.** The quickest way to lose your fears is to join forces. Joint forces unlock the inner beast. What scared you by yourself becomes a rush within a group.

Teams re-define fear. The timid and the weak transform themselves through a connected central source of power. Perception changes, focus changes. What once made you flee now makes you fight.

- **Hotspot.** Teams provide wireless connectivity – energy transfer. Air quality is not a hoax; it's a real issue with serious consequences associated with bad air. Clean air energizes. Air pollution creates an environmental disaster that leaves you with a mess to clean up. But a dynamic team produces electricity that can pump up what you can't on your own. There's a limitless energy source deep inside but you have to plug into it. Getting plugged-in inside starts with getting plugged-in outside.
- **Connected souls.** Getting knocked on your ass is a fact of life. Happens in the gym, on the field, on the streets, in board rooms – no place is exempt from the threat of getting flattened. The biggest challenge in life is lifting yourself up after a colossal fuck-up. How we respond to a setback determines how far we go in life. Winning is easy to handle. Losing isn't. How we handle frustration, disappointments, embarrassment, failure, and old-fashioned ass-kickings make us or break us. Soul-lifting is the single-most important exercise in life. The greatest power of a team is the lifting ability of connected souls. Nothing matches the collective power source unleashed by a unified force that pushes and pulls in one direction. Souls of lifters, those who can pick up the knocked-down, experience the greatest reward in life – putting up ladders for others. The result is independence through dependence – freeing the soul by depending on each other.
- **Group armour.** Teams award a special uniform – group armour. You can't buy it. It has to be earned. Group armour is greater than the sum of individuals' armour. When aligned, group armour can't be crushed. The allure of group armour is a magnet.
- **Group mindset.** Individual iron-will is a force of nature. But group iron-will has a force of spirit that can beat odds that seem insurmountable. When iron-wills connect, individuals never mismanage the break point - giving up, surrendering, fleeing, freezing, disappearing, and quitting when the real action starts. Group iron-will breaks through adversity instead of breaking down. The reason is group mindset develops non-acceptance, referring to a refusal to submit to setbacks. Refusal to accept bad news. Non-acceptance is the most powerful fuel that drives through any barrier that gets in our way. Individuals who develop it won't be stopped. But only rare beasts can build it alone. The best way to build the refusal to crack at the first sight of blood is lining up together.
- **The law of demand and supply.** The most powerful force of a coach-led team is the unmatched quality of the performance demand. The true measure of a team is what is supplied upon demand. Calling out the inner beast is not an option to endure Athletic Darwinism. Calling out the beast is a survival skill – the ultimate self-performance demand. Flipping the switch that releases the inner beast is easier said than done. That skill doesn't just happen. Few people can learn to do it alone. A coach has to teach you how to do it. And your teammates have to enforce it. A CoLT-driven performance demand is a force of nature. A coach-initiated performance demand teaches you how to go deeper inside yourself than you ever imagined. And, peer performance demands make you go the deepest...to the core of your heart and soul, forcing you to find things that you would never have found alone. What is demanded is supplied.

What happens? What results from working out in a Coach-Led Team?

You are guaranteed to climb the ladder. You will stretch. You will reach higher. You will consistently keep moving to the next level. If you don't, the leader wasn't a coach and the group wasn't a team. It was a crowd – a mob.

The power of a team is limitless. Never underestimate the full force that of a team. It can unleash a fury that an individual might never experiences alone. Team training plugs you into the external source so you can plug into your internal source. The key to getting plugged in is directed reps.

Directed reps are the secret to growth, to staying in the game, to not quit at the first sign of mild discomfort, to not act like you're falling apart because of physical exertion, to cure work-aversion. Directed reps are forced reps – a coach forces you to do them when you can't force yourself, when your mind wins the battle of wills and you cannot force yourself to do what needs to be done. To make it, you have to make it happen first. But making it happen doesn't always come from within. The strongest external motivation is watching someone make it happen. The strongest inner motivation is the feeling of making something happen.

It's easier to go through hell with a team. Once you've gone through hell, you won't quit. Surviving hell sets your soul on fire. No clichés, no catchy motivational quotes, no bullshit...just enduring what you thought you couldn't.

Case Study #12: 90-10 Rule

The 90-10 rule. Well over 90% of the athletes I've coached made their greatest improvement during team workouts, training with a small group led by a coach, as opposed to working out alone. A team workout is organized, **structured coach-led training** with a clear purpose, strategy, and an active **Set-Calling©** coach who makes the calls during the training while working out with the team, not spectating from the sidelines.

Every athlete I've coached who has moved to higher levels was the product of CoLT – team lifting. Directed reps are the key to building the base -- a rookie lifter's fundamental mental and physical habits that will guide the shaping of a lifting career. The base habits make or break a workout career. 90% of what you will become, what you will look like, how you will feel about yourself all happen during the first 250,000 reps of your workout career. Quarter-million reps. That's how long it has generally taken my athletes to build a base that will last a lifetime. Rookies average about 100 reps in the gym per workout hearing my voice. That translates to about 25,000 coach's voice reps per year. During a typical 4-year career, they've heard me 100,000 times. Add at least another 150,000 reps on the-field and they have about a quarter-million reps of hearing and processing the same set-thinking message. The conversion from SET-thinking to set-thinking happens somewhere between 100,000 and 250,000 reps... where mind-**set** is build... iron-will mind-**set.**

The only problem with team listing is dependency *after* the lifter has built the base. At some point, every person has to learn to workout alone temporarily or fulltime. Isolated workouts have one distinct purpose – calling out the inner beast without any help. Learning to flip the switch alone. Building the automated switch is needed to survive the rigors of any type of manual labour. Learning to unlock energy and strength by yourself connects you fully to your own soul. A soul of a lifter is not fully developed until the soul can lift self and then someone else. Striking the balance between dependence and independence is necessary for continued growth. Total dependence means 100% reliance on a coach's **Set-Calling©.** Total independence is 100% reliance on self.

Every new level of performance has a base that has to be built. After the rookie phase of 250,000 team reps, the following is evident: Be coached when you need to build a base at any new level. Do it alone when you need to connect with yourself. Use *e***X***plode*, the **X Fitness System** and the **Set-Calling©** decision-making model to make the call for exercise selection, weight selection, workload, and intensity. How much to lift, how to lift it, the order, how many times, and when.

How to Lift Properly

S.E.T: Every exercise has a S.E.T.:

- **Stance**. The launch pad. The starting body position.
- **Explosion.** Liftoff. The first two inches of movement, and
- **Track**. The course. The natural path of the bar.

All three are connected. Stance determines whether there's an **explosion** or a sputter and whether you stay on course or crash. Bad form, bad results. No workout program exists that beats bad form.

The 90-10 rule applies once again, this time to lifting properly. During 42 years of working out, including the past decade as a gym owner, I have seen less than 10% of people lift properly. Over ninety per cent fail to lift properly and fail to lift to failure. Bouncing, jerking, swaying, yanking, slamming… erratic lifting – more symptoms of impairment than a drunk driver. Erratic lifting is both a waste of time and dangerous.

Learn to lift properly. The results of strict form are astonishing. When you're not making the gains you expect, do inventory of your form. You're guaranteed to find the solution by identifying and correcting unnatural form. It takes mental discipline to do things right every time instead of sinking to half-assed mediocrity simply because it's easier. Technique starts with **S.E.T.** – an alignment of force, a connection between body position, the first two inches of lifting, and the natural path that a weight must travel to build maximum muscle and strength.

Stance includes hand placement, feet placement, and angles of upper and lower body. You can't arbitrarily position your hands, feet, torso, and legs. Every stance is purpose-driven. There's a reason for every millimeter of separation between body parts and the angles of the lower and upper body. I am a tyrant about stance with my football players because on-field stance makes an impact. On-field stance determines how much force is delivered and received. Crush or get crushed. My obsession with proper stance extends to the gym. I have to build players' mindset about how and why things have to be done right. Habits are transferrable. The habit of doing things right in the gym develops self-discipline that transfers to all other aspects of your life. The willingness and capacity to do things right starts with iron-will mindset that directs the physical act. If you don't give a shit how you do something, it's impossible to develop hardcore positive habits.

The two-inch explosion is the liftoff, a transfer of energy that determines the quality and quantity of reps. How much you lift is directly connected to the power generated by the two-inch liftoff. The difference between building extraordinary and ordinary strength is the unassisted power invested in the two-inch liftoff. The power of the liftoff ensures the flight of the weight. No liftoff, no flight. The keys to building maximum two-inch liftoff are:

- zero momentum – use only the muscle(s) being trained, and
- iron-will – you have to call out the inner beast on every rep to recruit every fiber of mind and body muscle available to achieve the equivalent of liftoff combustion. If there's no smoke and fire on the two-inch liftoff, you're cheating yourself because of lack of will – laziness.

The liftoff is the first two inches of the track that extends from the stance. Every exercise has a track, a natural path that the weight must travel. The track ensures that the work is being done by the right crew of muscles while preventing injuries. Going off-track will not build peak strength or muscle. And it will land you in a doctor's office. Wrong stance side-tracks.

S.E.T.-thinking has to be replaced by set-thinking. S.E.T.-thinking is a focus on how to lift right – stance, explosive liftoff, and track. Set-thinking is a focus on calling out the inner beast during a set to get the most out of your power source. It's impossible to think about both simultaneously. It's either **S.E.T.**-thinking or set-thinking. **S.E.T.**-thinking will not bring out your best or your beast. Only set-thinking will.

S.E.T.-thinking is the result of:

- inexperience,
- bad habits,
- unconquered fear, or
- all of the above.

S.E.T.-thinking is not an affliction that can happen only to novice lifters with zero lifting experience. It can happen to any veteran lifter who enters one of the infinite next-levels. The goal is to make the transition away from **S.E.T.**-thinking to set-thinking. The answer is reps – thousands of reps – to build the neural pathways that iron out muscle memory. **S.E.T.**-thinking vanishes when lifting becomes an automatic, second-nature action instead of an active-thinking process. The reason is that consciously thinking about proper lifting promotes one of the worst-case scenarios – thinking about crushing fear. This can happen to rookies or veterans. The uncertainty and unfamiliarity of every new level brings the potential of a crushing fear that changes focus from set-thinking back to **S.E.T.**-thinking. It's impossible to make meaningful strides toward strength potential by actively thinking about how to position yourself, where to place your hands, how to start the lift, and how to finish it. There's only one type of thinking that will get you to the next level – set-thinking... calling out the inner beast.

Set-thinking is a one-track mind, a search engine that focuses on one objective – to go as deep as possible to release everything you've got stored up – fuel the fire. Yet, what you're supposed to think about during a set is the most ignored element of working out. It's not written about, not lectured about, not taught. Here's what I have taught all my players – **call out the beast**. But, 'calling out the beast' is an abstract concept and an outcome. It doesn't teach how to do it. It only declares what has to happen. It's not enough to simply growl, *"Call out the beast!!"* and then foam at the mouth, scream, and hope for the best. One of the secrets to any teaching and learning is ***change abstract language to concrete language.*** Concrete language includes a step-by-step procedure that leads to the intended conclusion.

Set-thinking (calling out the beast) is accomplished by building a performance demand. What you're thinking during a set has to constitute a performance demand. Otherwise, performance sinks below average; you'll simply go through the motions and barely get by. And it has to block out any other message the mind will send – temptations to give in to the stress and rigor of exertion. Set-thinking has to win the war waged in the mind, where two sides are fighting for air time. The inner clash. The great debate. To nail it, your inner dialogue has to be on the offensive, has to attack opposing thought, and has to make the performance demand win by dominating the air waves. The mind is a battleground during every set. Without a strategic plan, it will become a wasteland, a disorganized mess that will need major reconstruction.

There are five compulsory elements of set-thinking, the ingredients guaranteed to make a performance demand that will push you to the next level:

- Challenge
- Rush
- Make it happen
- Separate from rest
- No quitting, no escape.

A passion for the challenge is what flips the switch. A challenge triggers the choice between fight or flight. The decision that forges our identity – our personal brand. A chickenshit or a fighter. Whatever you chose becomes habitual. The secret to making the right choice is to change your attitude toward challenge. Need it and love it. Passion. All passions are developed one rep at a time by experiencing the feeling… one rep at a time. The feeling is addictive. The feeling is what gets you hooked to the challenge. That feeling is the rush.

A passion for the rush keeps the switch on. The rush is the thrill that separates living from being alive – having a pulse. Needing the rush is the high-octane fuel that changes mindset from fearing a challenge to inviting it. Contrary to popular myth, feeling the rush doesn't just happen. It's not guaranteed. You have to make it happen.

Needing to make it happen is the heart and soul of a beast – achievement-orientation. A craving for stretching past pre-conceived limits. Wanting to make something happen is nowhere near enough. Neither is wishing or fluffy positive thinking. A passion to make it happen starts very deep in your guts. It separates you from the rest.

Separating from the rest is the deep need to be different – to make an impact. Make a mark. To do something out of the ordinary. A refusal to assimilate into the mainstream of mediocrity, marked by bitterness and resentment of underachieving. A passion to separate from the rest will instinctively build a refusal to quit.

No quitting means "becoming an unstoppable force." No one is born this way. A refusal to cave in and crumble when your comfortable world gets jolted, has to be built. Running away from adversity is more common than standing up and fighting through it. The reason for a chronic soft, weak will is simple – conditioning. Poor conditioning. Negative conditioning. Being rewarded for not being accountable or responsible. Never having cowardice called out and kicked out. Never having to face consequences, accept consequences, admit consequences, and, being forced to fix them. Running away has one cause – the available escape – the one that was never closed. And the temptation to take the escape route was stronger than the will to reject it.

Editorial #7

One of the leading causes of habitually choosing the escape route instead of facing adversity is the side-effect of CheerLeadership. Cheerleading is a type of leadership that promotes quitting when things get too tough. Cheerleaders build quitters. Cheerleaders applaud everything – strengths, weaknesses, and everything in between without the courage or conviction to even try effecting change. Cheerleaders are coddlers who shelter and protect from Goliaths, from facing them, fighting them, or even acknowledging them. Chronic escapism leads to dropped weights without dropping weight. It builds a weak inner dialogue, one that promotes and rewards half-assed effort resulting in the low-maintenance program – born weak, stay weak. A passion to not quit is by-product of a true performance demand that closes every escape. If your inner dialogue does include or conclude the concept of *not quitting,* potential will never be realized. It will get locked up and buried so deep inside that it becomes corrupted – unrecognizable and unretrievable. Corrupted potential can be prevented by breaking the habit of quitting before you've spilled your guts to fully finish a job.

Become Your Own Communications Director

How do you compose your inner dialogue so it leads to performance demand-building set-thinking? How do you become your own communications director? How do you become your inner speech writer? How do you become a set-thinking specialist? A two-step process – hear it, repeat it. Step #1 is the outer voice – the coach's voice telling them exactly what to think during the set. Step #2 is the inner voice – the lifter's inner voice takes over after conditioned to do so. The transition from step #1 to #2 is not easy. It doesn't happen overnight. The outer voice doesn't get suddenly replaced by the inner voice. A gradual process blends the two until the lifter's inner voice takes control over the air time.

What do you say? Is there concrete content, a script that can be followed that works every time? There's no script, no formal language that fits every person and every situation. It can't be rehearsed. All inner dialogue has to be customized. Set-thinking is personal because it has to come ***straight from the heart*** and ***heard it from the heart.*** The heart is the source and the receiver. I have never met a rookie who can do it alone, who can make a full transition from S.E.T.-thinker to set-thinker. The solution is to do it for them, teach them using a point-of-reference – hearing it first from someone else.

What's the best evidence that S.E.T.-thinking has replaced set-thinking. Two types of evidence – physical evidence and statements. Physical evidence is performance. The lifter's performance will sky-rocket when thinking changes from fear-based to beast-based language. The best statement that proves to me that it has happened is, ***"I hear you in my head."*** I was told this four more times just this week by people I no longer coach – ***"I still hear you in my head."*** That's how I know it works. Hearing voices long-term. That's the biggest impact you can make – get in his/her head… and stay there. That's the secret to replacing crushing fear with calling out the beast.

Case Study #13: Right to Silence

Canadian police read a statement called a "Caution" to every suspect (for their own good). It's a warning not to talk. In the USA, it's called the "Right to Silence." I have my own caution for the gym:

"Don't talk to me during a set. Don't try to motivate me. Don't say a fucking word. Just shut the fuck up when I'm lifting."

Sounds rude but it's not. It's essential for safety – mine.

Most of the athletes I've coached share one thing with me – we had to be made. Like the vast majority of athletes I've coached, I wasn't born with natural athletic talent. I am not genetically gifted. I had to be built, put together. Learning to call out the inner beast is the replacement for natural talent. But, learning to flip that switch needs the work of a mentor. Mine wasn't human.

I have never had a strength coach. I have never been taught by any human being how to workout, where, or why. I have never been motivated by a human to workout. Never needed to be begged, pleaded, prodded, cajoled, or coerced to work out. I relied on my soul of a lifter and the energy bounced back by the souls of lifters I've been blessed to coach. I had to make the transition from S.E.T.-thinking to set-thinking on my own, long ago. My inner dialogue is well-developed – advanced. I don't need or want to listen to any person open their mouth trying to motivate me. There are two reasons why...two reasons that make all the difference in the world between ordinary, half-assed workouts and extraordinary ones, the memorable kind:

- The majority of people I have met have a hard time dragging their ass out of bed, off the couch, or out of the bar let alone under the bar. They can't motivate themselves, nevermind someone else. I have never met or coached or taught a powerful motivator. I have never personally met anyone who can genuinely motivate me in the gym. The people I train are amateurs as motivational speakers. Here's an example: Shorty after I opened my gym, X Fitness, one of my former players, turned competitive bodybuilder, asked me to train him. I thought he knew my rule to shut up while I lift. He forgot. His urging me to do more reps was the worst example of verbal communication I had ever heard. He sounded like he was gasping for air or suffocating – the typical bullshit that you hear polluting the air inside a gym. In those moments, it's important to tell the person to shut up before they ruin the rest of your workout. I did and that was the last workout with him ever. It's not worth sacrificing my workouts for a client.
- If you have an advanced inner voice, amateur motivators are major distractions. They will cut you off from your inner self, unplug you...complete disconnection. Your connection to your soul of a lifter is your greatest gift. There is nothing more powerful than a connection to a higher power. If you can't connect to your soul of a lifter, connect with someone else's until you get plugged into yours.

The business of developing iron-will mind-set is the hardest part of working out and the biggest coaching challenge without exception. Weak-will will quit. Find what's inside and get plugged in.

Zero Momentum and ControL.L.L: Cheating Won't Result in Failure

S.E.T. guides where the weight has to travel but not how. Like traffic laws, there are rules of the road that govern speed, stops, and erratic lifting. You can't drive like a lunatic and expect to arrive safely. Obey the rules of the road.

There are 2 rules of the road that prevent collisions and safety hazards — **zero momentum** and **ControL.L.L.** Zero momentum means no cheating – no excessive force to lift a weight. The proper use of force results in using only the target muscle(s) to lift a weight. It means staying rigid throughout the set – staying in your stance. No momentum from outside forces. No heaving, no yanking, no swinging, no swaying, no arching, no leaning.

ControLLL means strictly **L**ifting, **L**ocking, and **L**owering the weight. Full power over the weight. Don't let the weight control you – you control the weight. ControLLL is accomplished by following the speed limit. There are 3 phases to every rep of every excercise – positive, negative and locks...lock up or lock down. The positive stage is the upward lift. Up, stop, down, stop... constitutes full range of motion for one rep. Negative stage is the downward return of the bar to the launch pad. The negative stage can handle more weight than the positive – **think about that when you're tempted to drop a weight** without any resistance. Letting a weight free fall during the negative stage wastes 50% of the lift and the strongest part of the lift. Half a set. Half a workout. And you can't use the excuse that lowering a weight is harder than lifting it because it isn't.

Positive and negatives are separated by a distinct, momentary pause where the weight locks up, stopping at the top of the positive lift, and locks down, stopping at the bottom of the return. Locks are stop signs where the weight must come to a full stop for the briefest of moments. The style objective of every set is to replicate the rep – make each rep identical. Same speed, same track, same form. The key is the speed of the weight – pace.

Traditionally, speed limits are designated by two digits separated by an x; example: 2x2, pronounced two-by-two. 2x2 means 2 seconds up (positive) and 2 seconds down (negative). I never use that system for three reasons:

- I don't believe in different speed limits (eg: 1x1, 2x2, 3x3). I only use one. Same speed limit all the time;
- The speed I use and teach is not perfectly balanced. My positive speed is slightly faster than downward speed; and
- I never count the actual seconds and never teach anyone to count for one simple reason – counting would interfere with the conversion of S.E.T.-thinking to set-thinking. Counting seconds is a recipe for disaster. The right speed has to be natural. Automatic. Second-nature.

Zero momentum and ControLLL are connected. Zero momentum is achieved by the two locks – at the top and bottom of the lift – the stops separating the positive and negative. The stop cannot be excessive at either the top or bottom. Just a blink of an eye. A deliberate stop, not a parking and holding of the weight. And, no rolling – no cruising through the stop signs. Full and complete stop so that the weight is motionless for less than one second. Executed properly, locks will prevent any momentum and recruit all the necessary muscle and mind fibers to accomplish two objectives:

- hold it at the top of the lift, and

- generate the most explosive liftoff possible. Stops are essential to prevent the madness of the trampoline syndrome – bouncing the weight off bodyparts and contorting the body to generate momentum. Momentum is false power that builds minimum strength.

The two-inch explosion is the key to every lift. Maximum speed is needed – rev it. You can't gently accelerate. You have to floor it. Pedal to the metal. Zero to sixty in 2 inches. ***eXplode*** the bar don't just lift it. The 2-inch liftoff starts each rep. Its speed determines how many reps will be lifted. The explosion has to be a violent movement – a zero momentum push or pull that calls out the beast…every muscle and mental fiber, ever rep. When you fail to lift what you want to lift, do a S.E.T. inventory. Check your stance, your explosion liftoff and the track. S.E.T. inventory guarantees that you will find the cause of failure. Study the S.E.T. of each set. The biggest cause of failure is a weak liftoff. If you fail to lift your 1RM goal, or 5RM goal or 225RM goal, the reason is likely a soft liftoff on one or all reps. One weak 2-inch liftoff causes another….and another. But, S.E.T. is a chain of events. Liftoff is connected to both stance and track. Start your study at the center, the 2-inch explosion, and work outward to stance and track.

Natural speed is the objective on the way up and down. Natural speed is a pace that forces the most muscle and mind fiber to activate during the positive and negative stage of every rep. It's a speed between 1-second to 2.5 seconds. You don't need radar to measure natural speed. Just look at the muscle that's being worked – veins and fibers should be exploding. You can feel natural speed. On the surface, 'feel' is an abstract concept but here's how natural speed feels – resistance. Natural speed has to feel like resistance. It has to feel like work. There's a flow to natural speed. Tires spinning and squealing for 2-inches, a gradual and natural braking, that leads to a full stop following by a slower, consistent speed on the way down. Not free-falling, not crashing and splashing. Control the weight so that the weight lowers at an even speed, forcing every possible muscle and fiber to work.

Following an explosive liftoff, the speed will naturally and minimally diminish until the weight stops at the lock up unless you're lifting at the speed of light… lightweight. Lightweight is any weight that offers no meaningful resistance at any point of a 19-rep set. In other words, the natural speed of the positive stage is constant instead of starting intensely high and diminishing slightly and gradually to a full stop.

Forced reps: I used forced reps for over 20 years with moderate success, then I stopped. Forced reps are assisted reps accomplished by cheating – self-generated momentum, or manual-assistance – externally-generated momentum from another person's force, or both. The concept of forced reps is connected to the ***natural progression of a set.*** The chain of events that characterize one set. For example, imagine a set of 8 minimum reps. If the weight selected is heavyweight, there are 3 potential phases.

- Phase 1: 6 maximum strength reps. The first 6 reps are full-range, zero% failure reps. Failure has not set in. The speed of each rep is the same. The weight is under complete controLLL.
- Phase 2: 2 struggle reps. Reps #7-8 need a struggle because of the onset of failure. MMF doesn't happen all at once. MMF is a gradual process that happens where MMF develops, starting first in the positive stage. The onset of failure is the equivalent of adding weight. Fatigue makes the weight feel heavier. Stage one of failure is the 75-25 stage – 25% drop in strength that constitutes 25% failure with 75% strength remaining. I call this the break-point. This is the last place where you can break through failure because the break-point line

is the entry to lock-out. When you reach the lock-out stage, there is no excuse for dropping the weight. No excuse for failing to finish the positive part of the rep. If you do fail to lock out, do inventory of your mindset. A lack of mental strength is the only cause for dropping a weight after lifting it 75% of the way. The 25% strength decrease will not prevent a full range positive lift. It simply reduces the lifting speed – the struggle. The negative speed remains the same as the first 6 reps. 25% failure affects only the positive, not the negative. The second phase of failure is the 50-50 line – 50% strength, 50% failure. You won't break through this on your own. Assisted reps are needed. How much? Enough force to reach the break-point only. Stage 3 failure is the last stage – anywhere below 50-50. At this stage, you need assistance to reach the top. The only value of forced reps at this point is training the negative stage with overload. The negative stage doesn't fail at the same rate as the positive. Generally, it has 25% more capacity than the positive stage. You should be able to lower the bar after fully assisted positive reps about 25% more times past positive MMF. When you have reached your goal of a minimum 8 reps unassisted, you're at the crossroads.

- Phase 3: Crossroads. After 2 reps at 25% failure, you've reached a crossroads at the 8th rep. Either strength plummets downward toward medium strength (50-50 line), or you flip the switch, call out the beast and keep you strength constant at 25% failure. If your strength drops off, you will not be able to complete a 100% full-range positive lift. Assistance will be needed.

Are forced reps beneficial? Forced reps are a paradox. There are pros and cons to forced reps. The purpose of forced reps is to build momentum during the positive stage of an exercise – move an unmovable object. Forced reps compromise one of two elements of a set – form or workload time. In some cases, both. Cheating is momentum generated by self-movement that compromises strict, proper form and workload time, referring to the time invested in using maximum force to lift a weight. Manually-assisted reps doesn't compromise form but reduces workload time – the forced part reduces the amount of full workload invested.

Cheating is not created equal. Neither is manual assistance. There are many degrees of cheating ranging from negligible movements to violent gyrations. The same applies to manual assistance – a range of negligible force to literally doing the set for the lifter. The problem is trying to strike the balance. Forced reps often is a seat-of-the-pants winging-it tactic… either not enough assistance of too much. Striking the balance is the key. Generating the right amount of momentum is not as easy as it looks. Follow the guidelines above, in the "3 stages of positive failure." Experience is the X factor. Assisted momentum has to be natural, referring to a steady even flow until the weight moves on its own.

There are three perceived positives to force reps:

- **Partial overload** – A forced rep is not a full-strength rep. The lifter didn't lift alone. Consequently, a forced rep is a partial rep, a partial lift with more than 100% weight capacity. Partial overload means performing a percentage of the positive stage with more weight than you can actually lift with the hope of someday lifting that excessive weight on your own. According to conventional wisdom, if a weight is too heavy to do a full-range rep, then do a partial rep...an assisted rep.

- **Extending a set past positive failure.** Forced reps force you to work longer. Increased workload time is a powerful way to train mind and body. Longer workload forces the mind and body to adapt by *compensating*… building more strength for the anticipation of the next time when even more work is expected. When the body and mind are fully prepared for a long-distance run, a short distance is a breeze. Extending a set far past the minimum will make the minimum reps easier and easier.

- **Building a tolerance for heavy weight.** To lift heavier weight, you have to know what it feels like. You have to feel the next level before you can reach it. There are two ways to feel next-level weight. Forced reps are the equivalent of making the bar heavier without actually adding plates. The phantom extra weight corresponds to the percentage of failure. For example, 25% failure equals 25% more weight; 50% failure means 50% more weight. The first way of using forced reps is going past the minimum, after you have actually lifted unassisted reps. The second way is more dangerous – full set forced reps. Put more weight on the bar than you know you can lift and have your spotter force every rep starting with the first one. DON'T TRY THIS. DON'T DO THESE BECAUSE THE RISK IS TOO GREAT. I have done these during my first 20 years but I made sure I had competent spotters and safety racks to prevent the bar from crush my throat. In retrospect, I recognize it was crazy to do them.

The negatives of forced reps are:

- **You can die.** If you lose control of the bar, the weight will crush you to death. Your life is in the hands of your spotters. S/he had better be competent. Assistance needs competent assistants. Forced reps are high-risk. One slip-up and you're in the morgue or emergency ward. When you don't have 100% strength to lift a weight, you relinquish independence. Dependency can be dangerous when you don't know the full extent of weakness and strength of your spotter(s). For this reason alone, DON'T USE FORCED REPS.
- **Assistance cancels resistance.** No resistance, no explosion. Forced reps eliminate the 2-inch liftoff. The 2-inch explosion is the most important part of resistance training. No liftoff, no flight. Forced reps eventually become another set for the spotter, who ends up doing most of the work. The loss of liftoff reps adds up. Liftoff reps are one of the differences between average strength and beast strength. Every rep counts. Mastering the 2-inch explosion translates into force that ensures the weight's flight. Assisted reps negate the repeated practice of putting everything you have to drive the bar. Cheating and external manual assistance removes an essential strength-building element, an absence that will catch up to you.
- **Strain causes pain.** The risk of injury dramatically increases with forced reps. Lifting more than you can handle causes wear and tear on the body.

Here's my conclusion to my personal study of forced reps:

- All my 1RM, 5RM, and 225RM personal bests happened during my forced reps era.
- All my athletes' 1RM, 5RM, and 225RM personal bests happened during my forced reps era.
- All my lingering injuries happened during my forced reps era.
- I'm in the best shape of my life, now, without forced reps.
- Since my forced-reps days, I haven't worked out with a full-fledged certified beast. I coach beastlings...baby beasts and intern beasts. I love them all but I don't trust any of them as

spotters. My focus in the last 25 years has shifted to coaching underdeveloped rookies and novices. My interest in forced reps has dwindled as my coaching career and my distrust of potential spotters grew.

- Without forced reps, my endurance strength dramatically increased. I stay stronger longer and have become leaner through the use of forced-rep alternatives including the "1985" concept, longer workload-intensive supersets and mega-sets, and the concept of making heavyweight through intensity. I use the theory of fatiguing muscle so that the last 5 reps are my heavy 5RM set and my last rep is always my 1RM. Sets within a set. I've replaced forced reps with reps forced by will-power. I haven't used forced reps in over a decade. The only side-effect has been a marginal drop in personal bests but there have been no negatives, only positives.

Case Study #14: "1RM" Solution

The true value of 1RM is debatable. For the first two decades of my workout career, 1RM was the centerpiece of my workouts. Back squats, front squats, deadlifts, bench press, close-grip bench press, shoulder press, weighted dips, weighted chins, T-bar rows...even curls – **barbell and dumbbell**. I had a deep need to know how much I could lift for one rep. It was both a psychological and physical need. Knowing I could lift heavy weight built up more than self-confidence. It developed a type of fearlessness. Breaking 1RM personal bests was a unique sense of accomplishment that I could count on daily. A self-test that was as simple as sliding plates on a bar. No matter how frustrating or boring or routine a day was, a rush was guaranteed simply by laying down the gauntlet – to iron and to self, in that order. When I failed a test, I got a rush from being pissed off but knew I would bust my ass to get it done. When I passed a test, I got a rush knowing I would never be satisfied – planning ahead for the next goal. But either way, pass or fail, I learned to call out the beast. I learned the arduous task of going deeper and deeper, trying to tap into the endless source of energy and power we humans have when we're plugged in.

Is 1RM essential? 1RM may be the ultimate workout paradox. For every fan of 1RM there is a detractor. For every positive there is a negative. I've discovered the pros and cons by relying on 1RM and then eliminating it. Here are the conclusions of my 42-year research.

First the positives:

- There was a positive relationship between 1RM and 225RM. When one went up, so did the other. When one failed, so did the other.
- Added to high-set, high volume workouts, 1RM built XXXL heavy-duty body armour.
- Nothing teaches how to flip the switch better.
- With a competent spotter, you can turn a successful 1RM into assisted 5RM, a potent tactic that is guaranteed to build beast-like strength.
- With a competent spotter, you can turn a failed 1RM attempt to a successful one in less than 3 workouts because 3 negative lifts are guaranteed to make one positive.
- Habitual 1RM successes build iron-will faster than any other lifting strategy because of the high-risk challenge – crush it or get crushed.

Now the reality:

- Pain. Continuous1RM will wear and tear you down. Without proper recovery, it'll bust you up. I worked shift work for almost two decades – started in a flour mill during high school and continued it with the most absurd 3-shift schedule while in policing. Seven afternoon shifts, one day off, 7 day shifts, 2 days off, 7 midnight shifts, four days off. Then court at 10am when you finished at 7am, court on days off, and overtime with every major crime that had to be solved before returning to "regular" schedule. Sleep deprivation, protein deprivation, carb annihilation – the trilogy of muscle destruction. It was impossible to eat 6-7 protein meals a day. But, I religiously lifted 1RM. Never missed workouts no matter if I had only 4 hours of sleep.

Eventually, the side-effects of 1RM combined with the reality of earning a living became painful. One injury after another. Chiropractor visits became as frequent as my workouts.

- Contracted contractions. 1RM doesn't contract the muscle enough times. But, as stated, it has to be added into the entire body of work – total number of reps count in one workout.
- 225RM went up without 1RM. The best way to increase 225 reps is to lift 225. Even though my 225 reps increased during my 1RM era, 225 reps increased higher as I decreased 1RM. Moving away from 1RM focused my attention on 225reps. What you focus on will grow.
- 5RM is my new 1RM. Adding 4 reps to 1RM adds ups. Over a year, it translates to a minimum of 1,000 extra reps. Probably more. Additional heavy reps cut you up without sacrificing strength.

Now the conclusion:

I re-defined IRM – changed my perception. I re-defined 1RM as the last rep of any set right before positive failure. Regardless of how many reps I do for any set, the last one is my 1RM by virtue of failure. Fatigue makes the weight feel heavier. If you go to positive failure, the last rep is the equivalent of a heavy 1RM regardless of what weight is actually on the bar or belt and regardless of how many minimum reps the set called for. Here's what I do on every set – remind the lifter, including myself, that the last rep is a super-heavy 1RM – because it is. I have conditioned my mind to believe that the last rep is the equivalent of 1RM. It works. The whole point of 1RM is to lift a weight that can't be lifted again. Actual1RM is followed by positive failure – you lift your maximum capacity once and then can't do it again. The last rep before positive failure serves the same purpose – the last rep before positive failure provides the most resistance, just like an actual 1RM because it feels heavier than what's on the bar. Theoretically, every set has a 1RM incorporated in it. Change the mindset, change the outcome.

The biggest barrier to actual 1RM lifts is fear – anxiety, stress, tension, apprehension. A super heavy weight is like a nasty opponent…an iron Goliath. Fear hides reps. This means that fear of heavy weight or fear or exertion or fear of discomfort or fear of getting crushed gets in the way of getting the job done – any job. Any high-risk activity produces negative creativity – images of hell, worst-case scenarios. Forecasting the worst is essential to survival but how you perceive it determines whether you pass or fail the test. If you view it as a challenge, you won't get crushed. If you don't, you will get steamrolled. If you focus on the rush, you will fight through the challenge. If you don't, you will rush away from the challenge.

The "last-rep 1RM theory" has worked with countless rookie and veteran lifters I've coached through overcoming their fear. Once they realize that the last rep of every set is the same struggle as any 1RM, they become conditioned to handling the stress of 1RM and breaking through mental barriers that previously limited their strength.

If you're failing to reach 1RM goals, try consciously believing that every last rep of every set is 1RM. If you want to eliminate 1RM, try replacing it with 5RM…as a 5RM set or a longer set with emphasis on the last five reps.

Case Study #15: Hidden Reps

It happened again last night. I stood next to an athlete I was coaching as she bench pressed. She was ready to put the bar down at 9 reps. Three words changed her mind. *"FIVE MORE REPS."* She did four more unassisted. On the 4th rep, the bar crept to a near stop at the break point but she locked out on her own.

On the fifth rep, she lowered the bar completely under control – an unassisted negative. As she lifted that 5th the fifth positive, there was no 2-inch explosion – no liftoff. The bar slowly raised to midpoint as I put two fingers under the bar. I felt the bar slowing to almost a complete stop at the midpoint because she was running out of gas. With two-finger pressure, I assisted her to the break point and she locked out on her own. There are 2 points I'm trying to make:

Pay attention as spotter. Look for evidence....see the signs that call you to action. The most compelling sign is a struggled full rep – a near stop at the break-point followed by an unassisted lock-out. This means get in position to spot. The next reps will likely be a partial rep to the mid-point. You can see it and feel it. One-hand pressure is usually all I need to help the lifter reach the break-point so s/he can lock-out on their own. This type of assistance is a 25% forced rep. Only ¼ of the positive stage was assisted – 75% was unassisted. **The 75-25 ratio is the spotter's goal**.

Pay attention as a coach to an incomplete set. Every set has a destiny.[7] Every set has full potential. Finishing a set before its full destiny hides reps. Wastes reps. Buries them. An incomplete set is the equivalent of stopping before the finish line. It's an intentional abuse of potential. A crime against self. Coaches have an obligation to prevent it. My personal research shows one constant pattern – **people stop about 5 reps before the finish line.** Over and over again, for decades, I have done the same experiment and received the same results. As soon as I see a crime about to happen (killing a set in its prime), I yell three words: "*FIVE MORE REPS.*" Almost 100% of the time, the lifter pumps out five more reps – unassisted or assisted. The ultimate performance demand. Without this performance demand, thousands of reps would be lost. Wasted. Hidden deep inside. Saving them is accomplished by the power of paying undivided attention to another person. This is the secret to coaching success. What you focus on will grow. Especially humans.

Calculating the last rep is directly connected to an anonymous skill – fuel-gauge reading. Figuring out exactly what's left in the tank, so you know when to challenge the mind and when not to. Every set has a natural struggle and a rep-span. It's up to the lifter to determine the true length of the rep-span. It's impossible to calculate the rep-span with 100% certainty before the set because the mind's response to the stress of fatigue is unpredictable. Pressure fucks-up the mind. The inner calculator goes on the blink. Our ability to read our inner fuel gauge suffers from DUI – Deciding Under the Influence...of fatigue. An impaired mind generates erratic thinking. Impaired lifting isn't a crime, it's a reality... and a problem that has to be solved to keep moving and improving.

7 Arcaro, Gino. *Soul of a Lifter.* Jordan Publications (Port Colborne, ON: 2011)

DUI causes an impaired mind to jump to conclusions, making false reads of an empty tank long before the needle actually hits E. False reads result in a pre-mature end of a set, leading to hidden reps…reps that get buried inside, locked up, and unfulfilled. This is why scripted workouts don't work out. A rigid scripted workout limits performance by wrongly painting a finish line before the set even starts. The only way to break limits is to draw the finish line during the set. The secret is to keep pushing back the finish line – make the race longer. Don't hide reps – free them.

Calculating rep-span accurately needs two components: i) it has to be done during the work-out in conjunction with reading the fuel gauge, and ii) needs a strong mind to teach you how to read the fuel gauge without bias. A strong mind is a mind not under the influence of fatigue… an unimpaired mind - a coach who is not in the actual act of lifting.

The greatest strength of a coach is reading an athlete's fuel gauge. Here's how to do it: watch for the first sign of quitting and add five reps. My investigation shows one major conclusion in connection with fuel-gauge reading: a fatigued mind quits 5 reps before the real finish line. This means that the inexperienced, untrained mind hides an average of 5 reps per set. Hidden reps accumulate, resulting in a heavy weight to carry around inside. It's called unfulfilled potential. Underachieving. The pain of underachieving is worse than the pain of overachieving. The pain of failure is worse than the pain of going to failure.

Here's my coaching strategy that has worked 100% of the time: the moment I recognize a lifter's intention to quit, I make a performance demand – "FIVE MORE REPS." The same three words each time. Nothing else works. I don't use words such as:

- "one more rep"
- "come on, you can do it"
- various "obscenities"
- "you're an animal!!!"
- or, the most absurd one… "no pain, no gain!"

Intention to quit (IQ) is also called mens rea, Latin for 'guilty mind.' How do you recognize IQ? Physical evidence. Three symptoms:

- dramatic decrease in bar speed;
- words…outbursts masked as excuses; and
- facial expression – fear.

Putting on the brakes, whining, and fright are three sure-fire signs of quitting before the set has actualized and reached its destiny.

IQ is usually recognized during the positive stage of a lift. As soon as IQ recognition happens, I wait for the weight to reach point-zero – the pause between positive and negative stages and make the performance demand – FIVE MORE REPS. It's important to make the performance demand at point-zero to alert the lifter's minds that it's been caught before the weight free falls to the false last rep landing. Busted. The minds now knows it cannot bullshit the lifter. As the weight descends down the negative stage to the launch pad, I make the simplest of all performance demands – LIFT. One word, concrete, simple, no ambiguity. A clear instruction just before the 2-inch explosion. LIFT is the magic encouragement word that guarantees LIFTOFF. Never fails. Then repeat. FOUR MORE REPS at point-zero, LIFT at the launch pad. Continue until the real last rep. Why does this work? What you focus on grows. Paying undivided attention to a person is the greatest investment you can make. Being interested pays interest. Undivided attention changes behaviour.[8] A performance demand is a potent, concentrated way of paying attention. The power of focus is a force of nature and nurture.

What if you're wrong? What if the lifter fails before the 5th rep? Simple solution – force the rep with 25% assistance. The body and mind will not know the difference between an assisted rep and unassisted. Neural pathways will be forged regardless whether the rep is assisted or unassisted. New habits are formed. Farm animal work ethic develops. The switch gets flipped. The beast gets called out. Five-for five. Five benefits for FIVE MORE REPS.

After enough coached reps, the untrained mind becomes conditioned to make unimpaired decisions. **Set-Calling©** becomes clear. Weight selection becomes laser-like accurate. The mind becomes the messenger of truth. The last rep becomes fact, not fiction.

Ultimately you have to learn the art of self-performance demands. Here's how to do it: Internalize your coach's instructions, then when you're experiencing fatigue and your mind tries to convince you to end the set, coach yourself with three words – FIVE MORE REPS.

Left unchecked, people will hide 5 reps at a time. Hidden reps add up. They accumulate like a heavy weight. Buried-reps is the top-rated reason for underachievement. Wasting a set because of pre-conditioned weak-will is the leading cause of unfulfilled potential. If you're feeling the crushing weight of underachievement, do inventory of your hidden reps. Unlock them or find someone who will do what your will can't. Learn to make self-performance demands or find someone who can make them for you.

8 Tribute to a masterpiece, *The Hawthorne Effect*. A study by Henry A. Landsberger concluded that showing interest in workers makes a motivational impact. The term *Hawthorne Effect* is used to describe any type of short-term increase in productivity due to showing interest.

Case Study #16: Painkiller

Workouts are my painkiller. I avoid pain with the most intense grueling workouts that my mind and body can withstand. I work to avoid is the pain of obesity, the pain of not surviving the frontline, the pain of losing, and the pain of not having my teams prepared. I work out with minimum rest – between sets and days off. On the average, I take only 2 days off in a 28-day cycle. Often, I work on a streak to see how many days in a row I can work out without a day off. My entire system is based on painkilling. It's my primary motive – the driving force. Not trophies, not ribbons, not stages, not photo-shoots. Painkilling. That's what has driven me to work out almost every day of my life without excuses, without complaints, without a coach, without any human motivating me or inspiring me or pushing me. I have no capacity to be motivated by humans. That's not bragging or arrogance, just fact. I have no receptors that are stimulated by human words or actions. My only motivations are challenges. I am driven by fear of leading an ordinary life. I am profoundly susceptible to boredom. Monotony, and the potential of it, is my high-octane fuel. My mind can't comprehend wasting my life sitting on a couch watching other people live their dreams. Working out the way I do and how often I do is my anesthesia. Some people drink gallons of alcohol to numb pain. Others inject and swallow a wide range of narcotics for temporary relief. My addiction is the rush.

As you will see, the exercises I use are the basics. Nothing fancy. I believe in old-school, hardcore exercises because they work. I never invented anything on my list of sacred exercises. But, the psychology and philosophy of my system is different... extremely different. What's my evidence? Performance. I personally have not met anyone who has worked out continuously for 42 years naturally – I've never jammed a syringe in my ass or wolfed down bottles of performance-enhancing drugs. And I have never met a group of athletes who developed farther or overcame more adverse conditions than the ones I've coached. They did more with less – no multi-million dollar taxpayer-funded facilities, no packed stadiums, no spotlight, no limelight.

Case Study #17: Iron Darwinism

I own a gym but I refuse to be a conventional personal trainer. I have never advertized for clients, never asked anyone to let me coach them. Why? I drive people away. Every year without fail, well over 100 football players try out for my football team. About 25, 30 (tops), finish the season. Not because I cut them – they cut themselves. **Athletic Darwinism**. Football is not a top priority for many Canadian males. They love the idea of wearing team jackets, of talking tough on Facebook and Twitter, and painting murals on their body but they don't actually love paying the price of investing their heart and soul in gym workouts and on-field workouts. However, of those who stick it out...well, I'm blessed to have witnessed some miracles.

I have been badgered by cops and wanna-be cops during the past 35 years to workout with them. Way over 90% leave and never come back because the truth hurts – literally and figuratively. They follow a 3-stage pattern – stage 1: Blowing smoke up my ass...Awesome workout, best workout ever. Stage 2: Head-scratching whining and complaining...in the gym and to avoid the gym. Stage 3: Fail to Appear. Iron Darwinism. Survival of the fittest. Over 90% let the gym's natural selection process crushes them. Iron Darwinism isn't a danger, it's an opportunity to be one of the strong that survives. But to those who view the gym and hard work as dangers, Iron Darwinism is an elimination process.

Recently, at their request, I coached two grown men. Persistent pestering – I didn't recruit them. After 40 seasons of coaching, I thought I'd seen and heard it all. I was wrong. On consecutive days, I heard and witnessed new lows – next-level absurdities. Shocks to the system. Low point #1: After a month of sporadic absenteeism, the first guy hesitated on his second set of chin-ups. When I told him he was delaying the workout by violating the time clock between sets, he said (out loud, in a packed gym), *"The bar hurts my hands."* Low point #2: The next night, whiner #1 was disgusted with whiner #2 who "has to learn to shut up during his workouts" because whiner #2 shouted, "*Hurry up, let's get this over with.*" A soft mind calling a weak mind annoying. Both were fired for "**crying for help**." First they cried for help and when they got it, they cried for help. The definition of a gym crier...a person who publicly announces his weakness – like a town crier.

Part 4.2:
Applying the X System

Each element of the X System has been explained. Now, it's time to explain how I apply it.

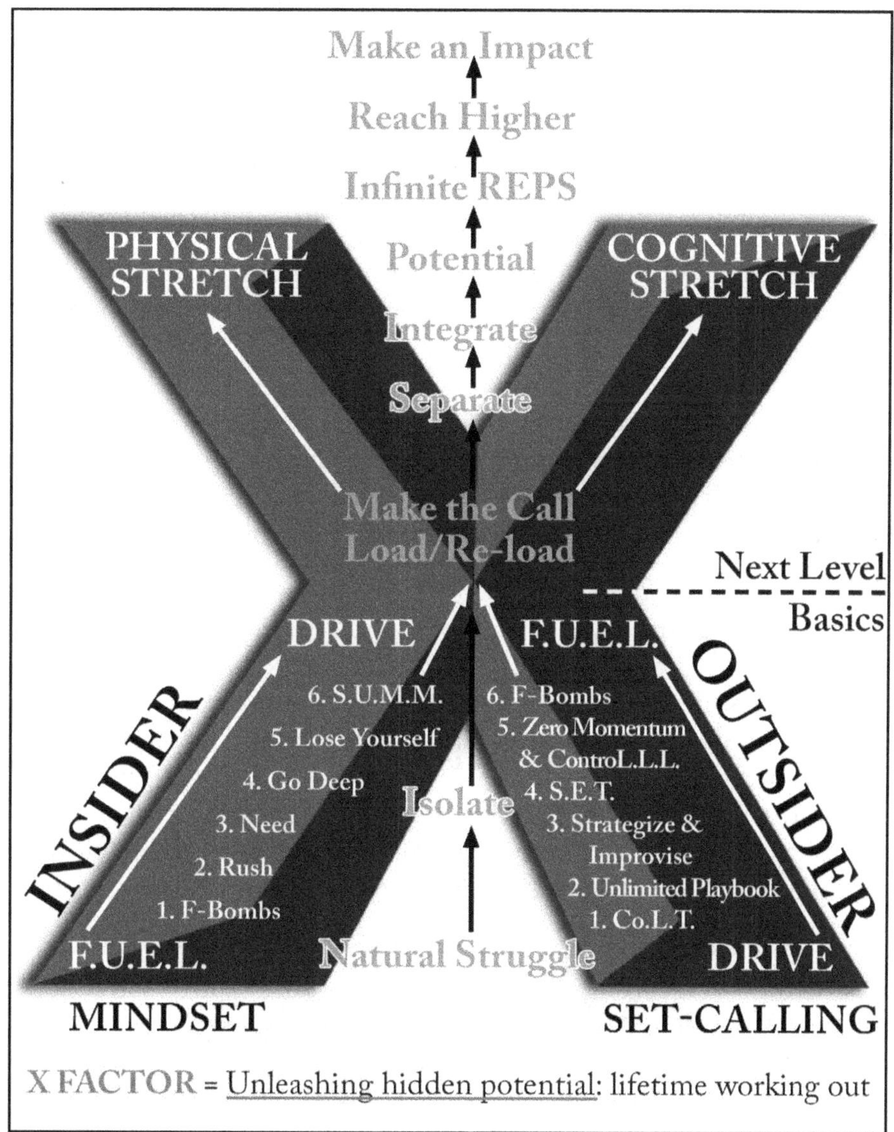

The letter X has four limbs – two on top, two on the bottom. Upper body, lower body. Two arms, two legs. They form two V-shapes, one upright on top, one inverted on the bottom. The connections are the important part – the union of the four limbs, two V-shapes. These connections tie together the **psychological, philosophical, and physiological components** needed to reach higher and move to the next-level. X signifies a power-build.

Applying the X Chart – key points:

- The goal of the X Chart is to demonstrate how to self-actualize by working out for a lifetime. To prevent early retirement from fitness and health, not to be satisfied with a brief workout career and then call it quits. Self-actualization does not have a finish line in your 30's, 40's or 50's, it doesn't have a mandatory retirement age, and it has no brake pedal. If you cross the finish line while you're alive, you have stopped living...you're just existing. Putting in time. Every human was created to build their gifts to their fullest potential. We were not assigned to planet Earth to take up space. There's more to life than reflecting on Glory Days.[9]

- Reaching full potential starts with mindset. Attitude translates to performance. Strong performance translates to tougher mindset. The mental and physical connection has complex dynamics but a simple approach – psychology and philosophy are the greatest influences on performance. Any performance – physical, intellectual, emotional, or spiritual. What we believe and how we think reveals in how we act, in what we do...and what we don't do. Nothing endures without ideological inconsistency. This means that although constant growth involves constant change, core ideology has to be consistent. We have to passionately believe in something to make things happen. That doesn't mean stagnation through blind conformity. We must question, challenge, and test our ideology to explore and expand who we are, what we're about, what we can do, what's stopping us, and what we have to do to overcome and break down our barriers. But we need passionate beliefs to fuel our drive. Passionate ideology, passionate performance. And vice-versa. Build your personal and team ideology. It's a work in progress that's constructed by fitting together one building block after another. Build your own culture of passion. It won't happen on its one. Left unattended, your personal and team environment will reduce to a culture of apathy, a toxic environment that promotes lethargy and leads to decay and decomposition.
- Reaching full potential requires a stretching program – physical stretch and cognitive stretch. Body and mind continual growth. Expanding past pre-conceived limits. The top 2 limbs (V-shape) represent physical and cognitive stretches to "next levels." "Next levels" are not neatly divided into beginner, intermediate, and advanced. Rookie, veteran, and expert are only general classifications of next-levels. There are steps within each general level but no concrete number of steps. The lines of demarcation may be clear or blurry because the ladder that needs to be climbed has an infinite number of rungs. There are limitless next-levels. The only limits imposed are by self. If you stop climbing, look inside for the reason why.
- Every next level has a basics stage and a lifting stage, Contrary to popular belief, the basics are not limited to entry-level novices who are beginning their fitness journey. The basic stage is a fundamental phase unique to that specific level. The significance of the basics stage is stability. A stable foundation has to be built at one level before lifting to the next level. Stability is achieved by ***consistent reps*** – reps emerging from similar programming, workouts that don't change in structure or sequence but change only in volume of reps and weight – to make the new level of performance second-nature. The lifting stage pushes you to the next level with ***challenging reps...*** reps that change in weight, volume, rest period and structure/sequence (changing workload, exercise selection, and order of exercise). The combined effect of consistent reps and challenging reps ***stretch you physically and mentally.***

In other words, the basics provide the launch pad for lifting upward to the next level. Once you reach the next level, the cycle repeats. The line between one level to the next is determined by new performance and growth. ***When you're doing what you've never done, you've crossed the line to the next level.***

9 Tribute to a masterpiece, *Glory Days.* By Bruce Spingsteen.

The basics and the lift stages are governed by the bottom of the X – the two legs. The left leg is the fuel that drives the insider…the 6-step psychology of iron-will mindset. The right leg drives the fuel for the outsider… the 6-steps of **Set-Calling©**.

The two legs converge to **make the call – load, then re-load.** Making the call is illustrated as the box in the middle of the X. It's positioned there because the calls are the result of the decisions made (as illustrated) by the two bottom legs: exactly how far you will stretch upward along the two arms of the V-shaped upper body of the X. Workouts are a series of decisions – how you reach them and what you do with them determines how high you reach.

There's a vertical path that splits the X from the bottom to the top. This is the V-path to potential. There are five boxes on the V-pathway. The first is natural selection. The objective of each workout is to make decisions that build resistance – a tough challenge… a natural struggle that will force free will to decide between getting stronger or staying weak. That decision is the secret to reaching your goals. If there is no natural struggle, weakness will be kept alive. The second box is **isolate.** Part of the struggle requires training without an audience and without the comfort of social connections. The third box is ***separate*** – separate from the rest of the competition. Move out of the congested traffic called the mainstream into a league of your own. Box #4 is ***integrate*** – coach others. Teach. Mentor. The greatest reward is putting up ladders for others. Making others climb makes you climb. Pushing others past their limits pushes you past your limits. Integration is a connection with other souls of lifters in order to unify forces in one direction. The 5th box is potential... another step toward self-actualization. One more step toward letting your full potential escape.

Part 4.3:
Sacred Exercises

"I fear not the man who has practiced 10,000 kicks once, but I fear the man who has practiced one kick 10,000 times."

– Bruce Lee

My Sacred Exercises is a short-list of exercises that I've made even shorter during four decades. The reason is ***REPxertise*** – to become an expert at anything, you need to do a decade of challenging reps[10] – the same exercise over and over again but heavier and more intense. More weight, less rest.

∞

10 Tribute to a masterpiece – *The Decade Rule of Expertise.* By Dr. Anders Ericcson. His published research in showed that expertise is developed by a decade of "*deliberate*" practice, referring to practice that is increasing challenging with stronger competition.

Case Study #18: Get Fired Up or Get Fired

Factory work was a miracle. Extreme manual labour changed my life. It transformed my body and my mind. It was a cure for teenage dysfunctionalism and obesity.

For my first three years of my workout career, I did only three leg exercises – back squat, front squat, and standing calve raises. That's it. That's all I knew how to do. I could barely bend over to tie my shoes because of my gut hanging so I focused simply on getting the hang of two simple up and down movements – squats and calve raises. Can't get much simpler than that.

As I started high school, I was blessed with a team of elite strength coaches – at the flour-mill – my foreman, my father and my co-workers. They taught me the secret to building raw, hardcore strength - **Mindset and Movement.**

Movement referred to the FOURce…the four forces of building muscle: **Move** something heavy, **lift** something heavy, **carry** something heavy…and **shut up** while doing it because you can't talk and work hard at the same time. Mindset is the blue-collar work ethic – get the job done, no excuses, no escape. Zero tolerance for the **L-connection** – **l**aziness and **l**osing. The blue-collar mindset gave only two choices – get fired up or get fired.

My strength coaches taught me that if you can consistently move heavy weight in 4 directions eight hours a day without cracking under the pressure, you will build the beast – inner strength, outer strength, you will get fired up, you will get the job done, and you won't get fired. The 4 directions are:

- dead-lift it upward, off the floor
- clean it upward, to your chest
- squat & press it upward, overhead
- carry it forward, on your shoulder.

My training philosophy and workout psychology were formed. My list of Sacred Exercises was built. So was my teaching-learning progression. Squats (back & front) and standing calve raises first. Do no other leg exercises until REPxertise if developed. Then add other exercises. Get really good at the basics first. Fundamentals build the mental and muscle base. From my first workout as an obese 12 year-old to last night's workout 42 years later, I have never abandoned my Sacred Exercises or my teaching-learning sequence. Nothing endures without ideological consistency. Core beliefs makes anything last.

Case Study #19: Does it Work for You?

Great coaches don't have to actually coach you on the field or in the gym. They can simply teach you one lesson that will stay with you for life – a voice that stays in your head... even if it's only one line. In the offseason following my 1984 rookie head coach disaster, I attended a coaches' clinic. A university offensive line coach lectured about blocking, the fundamental skill that protect ball-carriers from getting killed. He was brilliant. He taught a step-by-step concrete teaching plan – blocking for dummies.

Three days later, I phoned him. I introduced myself as JUST a Canadian high school coach. He said, *"Don't say JUST. You're doing one of the most important jobs in society. Probably for next to nothing."* Actually, for free. With 18 words, he transformed my mindset. Nothing has had a greater influence in shaping my coaching philosophy. Regardless, I still asked him my question. I explained a blocking technique I had developed for the center position, the guy who has to snap the ball to the quarterback to start every play. The center has a tough job – one of his arms is occupied with the snap but he has to recover quickly and use both arms to block a nasty defender who intends to rush at, hunt down, and flatten whoever has the ball. After I passed my idea by him, he asked a question... one that simplified my life: *"Does it work for you?"* Yes, it did. In spring practice, the center was actually winning the battle of the trenches. The simplicity of his wisdom hit me with the force of a quarterback sack.

What does this have to do with working out? Two things. First, if what you're doing works, it's a great system. Find what works for you, believe in it, ingrain it into your philosophy, and then trust it. Be ideologically consistent. Nothing endures without ideological consistency. Secondly, you are not *just* a lifter and you're not *just* a strength coach and you're not *just* a fitness instructor. You are making an impact on yourself and others.

The strongest evidence that something works is performance. If it gets results, it works. If it achieves what you set out to do, it works. If it's winning, it works. Simplicity, by its nature, is so unassuming that it's easy to ignore it. Simplicity is practical but not sexy so we look for something more glamorous. ***"Does it work for you?"*** has stuck in my mind ever since. It has become part of my decision-making process. I never spoke with him again until twenty years later when David met Goliath. My brand new Canadian collegiate team played his American legendary program in our rookie season. He interrupted my post-game speech with his, leaving me speechless.

None of this happened by coincidence. It was meant to happen. He could have not answered the phone, or let it go to voice-mail and never have returned my call, or simply hung up on me for wasting his time. Instead, took the time to listen and send me the message I was supposed to hear. Thankfully, I invested money into a long distance phone call and thankfully, I listened to 23 simple words instead of ignoring them.

Case Study #20: Strength of Conviction

We hate what we fear. We despise what we don't like. We label what is too hard to do as being unnecessary, useless, and valueless so we can avoid doing it. So, we drop what's too difficult because we're lousy at it or because it causes too much discomfort.

A lineman I coached for two years on my collegiate team, asked me for help to get a pro tryout. I contacted a general manager of a pro football team to make a case for him. I sent the GM the player's athletic resume and game-video that provided evidence of a beast – a strong, lightning-quick nasty lineman. I also told the GM the truth, alerting him that the player had missed several weeks of off-season workouts because of uncharacteristic laziness, resulting in a rapid decline in his 225 testing for bench press and squats. The GM agreed to give the lineman the chance of a lifetime – an interview and tryout…an opportunity to get paid serious money to play a game that millions of kids have played for free, an addictive game. A chance that most people don't get leaving them haunted by the reality that they never hit it big…never made it to the big leagues.[11]

The GM cordially invited me to the practice. Open-access. On the field, in the gym. Ask anyone anything. Typical of the football culture; information sharing is run-of-the-mill. Secrets are shared, they're not kept secrets. I met with the strength coach who asked me if the bench press was included in my workout program. "Of course," I replied. "They're right up there with squats." Not knowing where he was heading, he announced, "We don't do bench press. We don't need it. You should get rid of it." Then he moved on to his plyometrics program.

If I had **never** heard, *"Does it work for you?"* I probably I would have believed that the bench press wasn't needed in football and scrapped it. I likely would have succumbed to blind conformity and taken out the bench press, a decision based in strong evidence – because the strength coach received a paycheque from a pro team. Among the valuable life lessons I learned as a police officer was to *evaluate* credibility instead of *awarding* credibility automatically because of a title. As a child, I had it hammered into my head that I had to believe all professionals – doctors, lawyers, teachers, cops… never question them because, well, they had titles. My parents believed in the presumption of competence. Fortunately, policing dispelled that myth, teaching me that evidence trumps presumptions that are linked to titles.

I kept the bench press. It stayed on my Sacred Exercise list because of overwhelming evidence that it works. There's a direct correlation between 225RM bench press and reaching the next level. Not one player I've coached reached the next level with a weak 225RM bench press – not just football, hockey, MMA, and bodybuilding… even law enforcement. Scrapping bench press would have violated the sanctity of a Sacred Exercise that made the cut based on hard evidence. Strength of conviction.

The lineman got cut. He didn't make it. The reason was weak upper body strength. He got pushed around and pushed no one around. He never got another shot. *"I really blew it,"* he said. *"I took too much time off the gym because I had to work. I just had a kid."* Just another example

11 Tribute to a masterpiece. *Big Leagues*. By Tom Cochrane and Red Rider.

of crying for help then and then crying for help.

Coaching moment: *"Using children as an excuse to not work out is a travesty. Using work as an excuse to retire from working out is ludicrous. Both are masks for a deeper problem – laziness. There's 168 hours in every week and you can't invest 4 hours to workout?? You waste that much time punching a keyboard texting and posting and reading bullshit on Facebook and Twitter. You waste more than 4 hours a week watching TV. You had the chance of a lifetime. You asked for help but you didn't help yourself. Remember this later on life. Don't ever turn you back on anyone. Put up a ladder for someone just like the ladder that was put up for you."*

When a ladder is put up for you, climb it. Opportunities don't just happen. Someone was called to make it happen. Opportunities, like genetic blessings including size and speed, are gifts from God that must be honoured. But we all blow opportunities. The key is to say, *"Never Again"*... and mean it. Repeating past mistakes is the only type of negative reps that don't work.

Don't ignore simplicity – Quality trumps quantity. A chosen few Sacred Exercises is far better than a playbook of hundreds and thousands of exercises. Here's why:

- Steep learning curve. It's easier to become an expert lifter at a chosen few Scared Exercises. Every exercise has a steep learning curve. Contrary to popular belief, you can't just pick up an exercise right away and master it. Every exercise has a unique technique that takes significant reps to master. Bouncing around from new exercise to new exercise keeps the lifter in a ***constant rookie-learning mode***. It binds them in the ***Lifting101 stage***. Every exercise you add represents a new learning outcome. A structured teaching/learning progression is needed to add exercises only after the previous level of exercises have been mastered. Otherwise, you remain an amateur at a large group of exercises instead of a professional at a smaller, chosen few group of Sacred Exercises.
- Evidence. 100% per cent of the athletes I've coached have transformed mind and body with a simple list of exercises. Simplicity has been the secret to their mental & muscle makeover. The same applies to me. I'm stronger and leaner at 54 years of age than at any point of my life by simplifying my list of Sacred Exercises even more than ever. The simpler and shorter the list the better. There is no need to have a huge playbook of hundreds and thousands of exercises in order to build the beast.
- Ideological consistency. A concentrated list of Sacred Exercises demonstrates ideological consistency to yourself and your team. It shows that you believe in something as opposed to a grab-bag of hits-&-misses. Nothing endures without ideological consistency. Neither will your workout career. Jumping around from new exercise to new exercise without purpose is a sure-sign of ideological inconsistency. Ideological consistency does not mean close-mindedness. It means find your core beliefs. **Investigate, find evidence, build the inner core of a rock-solid foundation for your system.** No system, no results. A system is a structured way of replicating high-level performance each time - not once in awhile... each time. A system is an assembly-line that builds the same high-quality product without fail. The efficiency of any system depends on how strong you believe in it.

- Change-ups are not motivators. There is no need to "change it up" to keep interest high. There is no connection whatsoever between "changing up" exercises and lighting the inner fire. The drive to work out for a lifetime is not linked to "changing up" exercises to stave off boredom. The definition of boredom is the absence of challenge. The secret to growth is increased challenge, not quantity of exercises. If new exercises are needed for motivation, immediate inventory is needed to check and fix faulty mindset. Getting bored of basic exercises that work is a sign of a weak mind...the inability and unwillingness to focus on the fundamentals. The desire to "change-up" exercises is a cry for help to escape the necessary struggle of doing ***basic reps***, a rationalization, a false justification that makes the soft mind justify not doing the heavy lifting of basic exercises.

"Muscle confusion" leads to mental confusion. Instead, I have stuck to the basics while ***changing the look of the basics.*** This means I change the concepts – amount of weight, sequence, total workload, rest between sets – but I stick to my Sacred Exercises. The key is adding stress... add more resistance, add more pressure because the body will adapt and compensate to greater stress. The body re-builds and re-constructs itself with muscle instead of fat in anticipation of more stress. Blasting the body with more work and harder work is the change agent behind the much sought-after transformation. Workload is connected to quality of exercises not the ***quantity*** of different exercises. Amp up the nature of the challenge but keep the challenge itself simple. The body will stop growing only when it gets used to the exact same workload but not to the same exercises ***if the challenge changes.*** Same exercises build neural pathways but they don't stagnate. Don't try to be good at hundreds of exercises – be great at a chosen few. It's easier to increase the challenge with the chosen few instead of trying to figure out the technique for countless exercises. Find what works and keep working it... harder.

Don't ignore simplicity is the governing force behind everything I do. I learned that this rule works and applies to every career I've worked in. Simplicity is the secret to success in policing, football coaching, college teaching, business, writing, and working out. We humans have a tendency to complicate everything we do because it makes us feel smart and look smart. Complicating a simple job is human nature. It's part of the approval junkie that hides inside us, waiting to jump out and show its face.

Part 4.3.1:
Chest

CHEST

*** Bench Press**

Hammer Strength Incline Press

Hammer Strength Decline Press

Dumbell (DB) Hammer Press

DB flyes

*** Pushups**

I have reduced my list of chest exercises to these 6. Bench press and pushups have been Sacred Exercises for my entire 42-year career. The reason? Nothing is simpler, nothing works better, nothing builds a stronger base. The simple act of pushing weight upward is life-altering. Pushing heavy weight up has been directly responsible for transforming chronic losers to winners.

As explained in Part 1, my investigation has found a 100% relationship between bench press and winning – when my teams bench heavy, they win big. Championships and perfect seasons are directly connected to 1RM, 5RM and 225RM bench press scores. When the core of my team reaches big numbers for all three bench press tests, I can predict with full confidence that we will pound the shit out of any opponent, anywhere, anytime, because of the **armour-effect**… bench press builds top-grade physical and mental armour. Armour to beat whoever lines up against you on the field or in real-life.[12]

The psychology of bench press is Darwinistic – crush it or be crushed. The act of pressing potentially crushing weight is symbolic. Unless you learn to handle resistance, life will crush you to the ground. Every day, the odds get bigger, barriers get stronger, mountains get higher. If you don't learn to smash the odds, even the odds will crumble you to pieces. The feeling of beating what was deemed and seemed to be insurmountable odds is the secret to building the confidence needed to enter the most dangerous stage. Whether it's a violent sport or the streets or starting your own business or writing a book or doing anything that risks what you have and tests the size of your balls, the difference between those who do and those who don't, between those who can and those who can't, and those who will and those who won't because they

12 Tribute to a masterpiece, Ephesians 6;11-13. "*11 Put on the full armor of God, so that you can take your stand against the devil's schemes. 12 For our struggle is not against flesh and blood, but against the rulers, against the authorities, against the powers of this dark world and against the spiritual forces of evil in the heavenly realms. 13 Therefore put on the full armor of God, so that when the day of evil comes, you may be able to stand your ground, and after you have done everything, to stand.*"

are too terrified to even try, is state of mind. Iron-will mindset will drive you onto any stage. Weak-will makes you run from it.

The secret to surviving any danger, anything that scares us, is **REPS** – **R**epeated **E**xposure to **P**ressure & **S**tress. Calling out Goliaths repeatedly. Standing up to monsters brings out your inner beast.[13] Every walk of life has monster pressures and stresses waiting to crush you. Each one has to be met head-on. You can't turn and run, you can't take detours to avoid life's struggles and expect to get stronger. Handling pressure doesn't just happen. It has to be developed. Depressing and pressing an Olympic bar with more weight than you weigh is guaranteed to build transferrable confidence that lets you crush pressure before it crushes you, in or out of the gym.

No job I've had is tougher that preparing someone's loved one, their pride and joy, their blessing from God Almighty who can't even shave yet and doesn't have a driver's license, for the violent world of football. Or, for the dark side of planet Earth called frontline policing. I've had no greater challenge than training someone else's children to survive what can kill them. The job carries a professional and moral obligation to teach them how to survive a type of punishing Darwinism that will steamroll the weak to make room for the strong to move ahead. My top priority has been to start at the top – build iron-will mindset. Psychology always beats physiology. All the natural talent in the world won't save you if your mind is unnaturally weak. I have found nothing that starts the process better than teaching student-athletes to hold a weight over the chest, lower it, and make a choice – ***eXplode*** it off the chest or let it sink the chest. Bench press is the ultimate exercise of free will. Lift your burden or let it depress you. Bench press has been a miracle transformation for myself and countless people I've coached. Bench press played the biggest part in unfuckulating my fucked-up 12-year old self, a socially, physically, and emotionally inept wreckage. An obese, dysfunctional child who never stood up to any of the long line-up of bullies, adult and adolescent, who targeted fat, weak kids knowing that the bullying would be uncontested. Google "bully synonym" and you'll find "***asshole, chickenshit, low-life, scumbag, gutless, no-balls.***" But there's a cure for a bully – call out the beast. When you transform self, suddenly your environment cleans up.

In my experience, nothing cleans up your environment better than challenging yourself with daily doses of iron. Iron detoxifies. An iron cleanse purifies your inner and outer environment. Your outer environment suddenly is purged of bullies. Nothing is more intimidating than watching someone press monster weight or seeing its by-product – chest armour. The pretend monsters go away. To be a beast, one must build the inner beast and call it out. Hearing what your opponent can bench for 225RM or 1RM or eye-witnessing it is depressing. That's why it's important to broadcast test results – websites, Youtube, newspapers…send an iron-clad pre-game message. Operation mindfuck.

Bench press and squats are tied for top spot of best ways to start immediate environmental clean-up. Although they are tied for first place, I've learned the best training sequence – hook 'em with bench press first, squats will follow. I don't mean ignore squats until bench pressing becomes proficient. I include both in every rookie program. But my investigation shows compelling evidence that bench press achievement lights a fire that carries down to squats – not vice-versa. As soon as a lifter ***feels*** the rush of successfully pressing more and more weight, s/he learns to flip the switch for every other exercise including squats. Bench press success breeds squat success. The reason is the degree of fear – squats are uncomfortable for rookies but bench press scares the shit out of them. Learning to bench press is an exercise in fear management. Squats can't crush your throat and kill you. Bench

13 Tribute to a masterpiece by Friedrich Nietzsche: "*Whoever fights monsters should see to it that in the process he does not become a monster.*"

press can. Higher risk, higher reward.

Can you get stale or bored of bench press? Not if you get addicted to the rush. I have never abandoned bench press at any time during 42 years of working out. I have never trained any athlete for any sport or any profession without including bench press. And never will. My motivation is simple – fear of losing the rush, fear of weakness. The two are connected. The rush of 225RM or 5RM or 1RM is addictive. You'll never get bored if you get hooked.

Like squats and carrying 140-lb flour bags, bench press is a consciousness-lifting exercise. My coaching objective starts with lifting levels of consciousness past the restriction of unmanaged fear. Any physical competition against the inner and outer opponent moves us up the scale toward higher consciousness, rep by rep. That's why bench press and squats are psychologically connected to winning and losing

No machine replaces the effect of an Olympic Bar and free weights. But, Hammer Strength bench press is the best "machine"...the best alternative that most closely duplicates the real thing. I started using Hammer Strength bench press to supplement free weight bench press for three reasons:

- safety, when no spotter is available;
- keeps me on track. Hammer Strength is engineered to duplicate perfect reps – every track is exactly the same. This lets you focus100% on the heavy weight; and
- to prevent more injury caused by my stupidity of wrong hand placement during my early years of bench pressing. During the past decade, Hammer Strength has never caused one injury. And my old ones have healed.

The secret formula to bench heavy is to bench press a lot. Consistency. The litmus test is 100 minimum bench press reps per chest workout. That's the line of demarcation that separates wanting it and needing it. Using this formula, not one athlete I've coached has failed to consistently improve both 1RM and 225RM test results – 100% success rate. No one has regressed.

I have never taken more than three consecutive chest workouts off from bench press. On the rare occasion that I replace bench press for more than two workouts, my mind plays games – I feel weak. Conservatively estimating, I benched my 500,000th rep four years ago at age 50. As a teenager, I formed three goals – bench 300 for 1RM, then bench 1RM for double my bodyweight and then bench 225RM for 30 reps. It took about 52,500 reps to crack the 300 lbs. barrier at age 17. About another 10,000 to bench 340 at 18 a week before I got hired as a cop. Then, it took me nine years to add fifty pounds – I benched 390 lbs. 1RM – over double my bodyweight (190 lbs.) at age 26. That same year, I benched 225 lbs. for 26 reps. I became obsessed with cracking 400 – never happened. 385, 380, 375 back and forth. But each 400 attempt ended up with a crash landing. Never equaled my 390 personal best either. And I failed to reach my goal of 30 reps at 225. Never broke 26 again. I equaled it in every decade but never broke the barrier. The good news is that it took only 145,600 reps to get my personal bests naturally. The bad news is that about 350,000 more reps haven't been enough to pass them. And, I've needed 350,000 reps just to maintain the exact same strength every decade without steroids. I peaked at 26, after 14 years of consistent lifting. But the best news is that I have never regressed since then. I stayed at my peak for another 28 years. At 54, I am in better shape that I was at 26 without any loss of strength. And no player has out-benched me during a workout. The head coach holds all team records.

Case Study #21: The Hurricane Effect

During my unsuccessful quest for 400 1RM and 30 reps at 225 lbs., an unintended positive happened from that negative. Set #2 became the growth set, the set where the most improvement happened…where performance stretched the farthest.

Below is an illustration of the stretch program that worked for me to reach my current personal bests:

Diagram 24

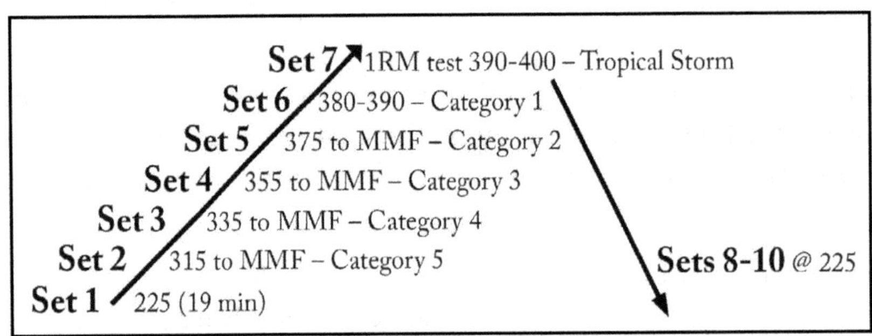

- This V-graph includes two tests – 1RM at the top (set #7) and 225RM at either set #8, 9 or 10.
- After a set of high-rep bodyweight pushups (unweighted), Set #1 was always a high-rep 225RM set, 19 reps minumim. Had to crack 20 reps – non-negotiable.
- Set #2 became the 315RM set…three 45's each side, to MMF.
- Sets #3-5 were each heavier by 20 lb increments. All three to MMF.
- Set #6 was the penultimate set – the set directly preceding the 1RM test. The weight selection ranged from 380 – 390. This range was elected based on the past – I had lifted it before.
- Set #7 was the test range, where I would either break my personal best or duplicate it.
- Sets #8-10 were fixed at 225. The goal was to break a personal best at one of those sets. Three chances to break the record.
- This stretch program had always worked for me and my players to reach personal bests – until I set the 400 1RM and 30/225RM goals.
- There are two relationships that govern all workout programs:
  - relationship between weight selected and the 1RM stretch goal, and
  - relationship between bodyweight (BW) and weight lifted (LW).

The stretch formula I use is a weight selection decision. It's based on *percentage of weight selected in relation to the stretch goal.* This formula is called <u>% Stretch Goal (SG) Range.</u> This formula selects weight by percentage of the 1RM stretch goal. Each set is governed by a percent range, e.g., 50%-60% of the stretch goal.

The best 7-set range is a growth from 50% of the stretch goal to 100% (the actual 1RM goal) on the seventh set. The 'actual %' (Column 2) was the specific percentage of stretch goal I used at each set to reach my personal bests of 390 1RM and 26/225RM.

Column 3 shows the ratio of bodyweight to lifted weight (BW/RW ratio). Column 4 is another way of expressing Column 3 – percentage of bodyweight lifted (%BWL):

Set #	% SG Range	Actual %	BW/LW ratio	% BWL
1	50-60% SG	58% SG	1.18x BW	118%
2	75-85% SG	81% SG	1.85xBW	165%
3	85-90% SG	86% SG	1.76xBW	176%
4	90-95% SG	91% SG	1.86xBW	186%
5	96-97.5% SG	96% SG	1.97xBW	197%
6	97.5-98.6% SG	98.6% SG	2-2.05xBW	200-205%
7	100% SG	100% SG	2.1xBW	210%
8-10	50-60% range same as set #1	58% SG	1.18xBW	118%

After reaching my current personal bests, this formula failed – but only on the back half of the graph. The front half still worked:

- Set #2 kept growing in reps.
- So did sets #3, 4, and 5. I increased the reps for each set.
- Set #2 grew the most in reps, followed by sets #3-5 in order.
- **Set 6 & 7 didn't grow.**
- Set 6 was successful at 380 & 385, but never again at 390.
- Set 7 at 390 or 400 never happened – crash landing…ZeroRM.
- Sets 8-10 equaled the past 26 but never broke it.
- The **"Hurricane effect"** – started strong as a category 5 storm, fizzled out to a tropical storm.

Conclusion: **Once you make up your mind to reach a stretch goal, a performance demand automatically follows that lifts consciousness level which in turn lifts the physical level which raises the bar.**

Failed stretch goals stretch performance. Fundamentally, the stretch goal is not the focus. The actual focus is the mechanism – the pieces of the puzzle, the collective steps of the ladder that you climb to get there. The stretch goal is a by-product. What you focus on grows. The real growth happens with each step of the ladder. In my experiment, the 2nd step grew the most. The second set at 315 more than doubled. The reps at third set and fourth set and fifth also grew – 335, 355, and 375 respectively. Rep efficiency during the journey. But rep deficiency happened upon arrival. The sixth and seventh did not work out like I had intended. Set six did not grow – it got stuck at 1RM or zeroRM. Set #6 ranged from 380-390. Sometimes I succeeded at 380 and 385 for 1RM. Sometimes I failed. But, I failed each time at 390. Never equaled my personal best again. Never broke it. The same failure happened during sets #8-10. My 225RM was equaled but never broken

What I intended to do didn't happen but what was unintended happed. The Law of Unintended

Consequences came into play because of intense focus during the journey leading up to the stretch goal. Initially, I wasn't aware of the unintended outcome. The obvious wasn't obvious. I overlooked the growth of set #2. Why? Tunnel vision. But as my level of consciousness lifted, the truth jumped out – ***stretch goal is actually a misnomer. It's the stretch ladder that counts. The stretch journey is where the actual growth happens.***

Pushups

The pushup is the only other lifetime Sacred Exercise that has made the cut since the beginning. Pushups are a bodyweight press. I do them unweighted or weighted (plate on my back) Whether on the football field or in the gym, I teach the psychology of pushups – the dual-purpose of bodyweight pushups:

- they train sustained workload – endurance resistance training, conditioning the body to deal with the discomfort of manual labour lasting more than a few seconds, and
- they predict and replicate bench pressing your bodyweight.

I teach my players to shoot for 30+ bodyweight pushups as *fundamental* mental and physical training to improve 225RM. High rep testing starts with mental stamina and fortitude – building mental fiber. Every high-rep exercise that ends in 5RM struggle on the last five reps does the job – it builds blue-collar work ethic, an attitude that breaks contempt toward physical and mental labour.

The way pushups are taught determines the return on the investment. ***Rep efficiency versus rep deficiency.*** Your attitude, how you execute, and for how long. That's the key to any exercise, any workout. And it's the key to applying strength. Strength is meant to be applied. I teach fundamental strength first, appearance second. I teach players to strive for high reps as a fortest – a test of endurance strength. I never use pushups as punishment or as time-killers. I use them to build stamina – mind and muscle stamina. The reason I emphasize endurance strength is survival. Two examples:

- Violent offenders sometimes resist arrest. When their switch goes on, they fight on pure adrenaline which allows them to fight for longer than they ever trained for. Bad guys don't adhere to a time clock. They fight for freedom. Until you've had to drag someone to a cruiser and try to force him into a car entrance that's smaller than him, it's easy to underestimate the amount of functional strength and stamina needed for personal survival. Cops get killed. That's a fact. That's reality. Violent offenders don't play by the rules. There's no magic training program that teaches stamina. Conditioning is simple – sustained workload. Exert yourself for more than a few seconds. Push yourself. Fight your brain. Beat the temptation to give up at the first sign of discomfort. Pushups do the trick. They are as good as any exercise to build funda*mental* strength and stamina.
- Violent sports like football last 60 minutes played over three hours. There's a myth that football training only needs short bursts of energy. Bullshit. Complete nonsense. A string of energy bursts over four quarters needs a lot more than training for short bursts of energy. I run a warp-speed no-huddle, the equivalent of high-speed interval training. Sprint, jog, sprint, jog…no breaks, no brakes, no down time. Even though pushups train only the upper body, they prepare the entire body for the mental and physical rigors of smashing into other bodies for three hours. Nothing is more embarrassing than a team than quits in the fourth quarter. Nothing is more humiliating than watching a soft, weak, out-of-shape, poorly conditioned team lay down before four zeroes are on the clock. I drill pushups every chance I can – in the

gym and on the field. We don't practice well-rested... we ***become*** well-rested by learning how to work like farm animals for sustained periods of time.

I got rid of pec-deck, cable-flys, barbell decline, barbell inclines, and dumbbell inclines and declines. I realized that pec-deck doesn't require gripping the bar. I never waste an opportunity to hold a bar to develop grip strength. Weak grip ends up in crash landings. It's impossible to lift heavy weight or use force in violent sports with soft hands. Cable flys aren't a compound exercise. You can't go heavy. They don't build functional strength. I stopped doing barbell declines when I realized the madness of lifting heavy weight while laying on a quasi-inversion table – focusing on not killing myself instead of the lift. Barbell declines are the most dangerous exercise known to wo/mankind. One slip-up and the bar smashes your throat. Barbell inclines did nothing that bench press didn't do.

Consequently I replaced pec-deck with a superset of DB flys followed by DB bench presses. This combination with zero rest blows-up my chest, grip, and forearms. I use them to supplement bench press – after or before. Fatiguing the chest before bench press is a fantastic way to make bench press feel heavier – resistance by fatigue – which adds reps and weight to 1RM and 225RM. I have replaced BB inclines and declines with Hammer Strength incline and decline. They're safer, allowing physical and mental concentration on a different press angles. Both are phenomenal ways to develop pure striking power, a survival skill for many football positions and techniques including blocking and shedding blockers.

The teaching-learning sequence has never changed – bench press and pushups first until REPxpertise is built. Then I add other exercises. Never have and never will mix other chest exercises with bench press and pushups until the athlete has become a competent lifter – a confident, fearless bench-pressing machine.

Chest conclusion: I have tried every chest exercise known to wo/mankind. My investigation revealed one simple truth – bench press is enough to build strength and armour to have prepared my students and myself for football and law enforcement. If you wanted to simplify your workouts and do just one chest exercise, get a flat bench, an Olympic bar, heavy plates, and bench press every chest workout. If you only did bench press, you would guarantee amazing strength, cast iron-will, and cast-iron chest armour.

∞

LEGS	
Triple Play	- Back Squat
	- Front Squat
	- Calve Raise - Standing & Seated
FOURce	- Deadlifts - Bent-legs, bar or flour bags
	- Hang Cleans - bar or flour bags
	- Bag Carrying
	- Squat & Press
Triangle	- Hack Squats
	- Leg Extensions
	- Leg Curls

The Big 10. These 10 Sacred Leg Exercises have been the difference between being fat and ripped, winning and losing, standing your ground and getting knocked to the ground.

Triple Play

Three of the Sacred Leg Exercises form the core… the ***triple play*** of my system – back squats, front squats, standing calve raises. No other leg exercise or combination has contributed more to the development of athletes from scratch… from point-zero upward.

It's impossible for a rookie to process and master every leg exercise all at once. I never have and never will include all 10 Sacred Leg Exercises to coach rookie football players or any other occupational rookie athlete. To build ***REPxertise*** I focus on the core. Every one of my athletes who has moved to the next level started with the triple play before adding the rest of the Sacred Leg Exercises. My investigation has found that the core triple play requires the least amount of skill, not to be confused with difficulty. Squats (back & front) and calve raise have been the simplest leg exercises for me to teach, the simplest for my players to learn, and the simplest to buy into. "Simplest" is relative. It doesn't mean easy, doesn't mean comfortable or relaxed. Simple means less complicated, less thinking, more doing.

The biggest workout mistake is neglecting leg work. Oddly, leg work doesn't have the same rep as upper body. It's not as sexy and glamorous as upper body is. Leg work is not an instant passion. Here's why – it's too hard. Leg work is extremely difficult. It's uncomfortable. Even painful. But, it's your choice – X or Y. Build a powerful X-shape with a V-shape on two powerful legs… or build a Y, a V-shape on a stick – and never wear shorts. And easily get knocked on your ass. Pain now or pain later. You can go through discomfort now or go through the discomfort of being horribly out of shape later.

As a coach, I know there are two secrets to developing a passion for doing leg work: evidence and addiction. Show them it works and let them feel the benefits. Then, get them hooked on the rush. I was lucky to have a passion for leg work from the start because my desperation – which was hanging around my gut – led to a performance demand. Obesity had interfered with childhood sports and was about to block high school football.

There is infinite literature that tells us about the virtue of goals. But goals alone won't score any points. Goals need bad-ass drive and determination to become an unstoppable force. If you can be stopped, goals are nothing more than entertaining anecdotes. A goal without fuel is running on empty. A guaranteed way to make a goal a reality is to make it a basic survival need. Once you need it that badly, like air and water and food and shelter, a performance demand will follow automatically from a place deep inside… from the soul of a lifter.

My first three years of working out featured only my core, just the triple play of leg exercises… with a bar, no machines. Out of necessity, I started with the lowest weight possible, high-reps (high-reps are an oxymoron for a fat 12 year old), and horrendous technique because my fat was getting in the way. My fat had no muscle. So I started with laughable partial reps. But, the Law of Unintended Consequences kicked in. Partial reps were a blessing because it taught me the value of ***breaking down a skill*** to manageable units – links of a chain. Instead of trying to learn the entire skill as a whole, get really good at each separate unit. Build the chain one link at a time. Eventually they unify into a force of nature. As it turned out, partial reps gradually progressed to full reps… naturally.

As the full reps grew, so did the H-bombs – hormone bombs. Squats flipped the switch, triggering T-blasts – testosterone blasts. High reps ignited GH-blasts. Add the adrenaline that goes with conquering a weight that is trying to crush you to pieces, turned into a rush… a monster rush. A consciousness-altering rush that got me hooked on leg work.

My passion for leg work climbed to a higher level at a flour mill, carrying 140 lbs. bags as my high school job. My foreman had zero tolerance for laziness. Performance demands personified. With support from my intolerant father who worked in the same place (who read me my "right to remain silent," and "the caution" to not get my ass fired or quit like over 90% of rookies who got crushed under the burden of heavy weight) I survived Occupational Darwinism. I beat the odds by making extreme manual labour a basic survival need. There were only two sets during the 8-hour workout:

i. 1200 reps of carrying 140-lbs. on your shoulder, and

ii. 300 reps of deadlifting and cleaning 140-lbs.

Every day. Fortunate for me, a veteran worker was assigned the job of teaching me lifting technique. He was a passionate, functional strength coach…. a soul of a lifter who broke down the science of functional leg work into simple components, basic easy-to-do fundamentals, all ending with the same instruction… ***"then, muscle it up."***

FOURces

It's amazing how the human mind will respond when you are desperate, when you have no choice about making it happen, and when you learn from a passionate soul of a lifter. I learned and repped out four movements (FOURces) in the flour mill that changed my life, by transforming mind and body with sustained extreme workloads that have to be experienced to be believed. Each one skyrocketed my gym leg work:

- Deadlifts. Deadlifting a flexible object (e.g., a flour bag) is harder than deadlifting a solid object (e.g., an Olympic bar). I was taught to do bent-leg dead-lifts to prevent debilitating back injury. I incorporated stiff-legged deadlifts in the gym during my high school career because of conformity. I thought it had to be done. In reality, bent-leg deadlifts with a pliable object has worked better for my athletes, building far more explosive leg strength than stiff-legged deadlifts. Eventually, I removed stiff-legged deadlifts from my own workouts. My flour mill deadlifting experience worked wonders for overall strength and made my gym deadlifts go through the roof. But they never out-did squats. Deadlifts packed on weight on both back and front squats but deadlifts never replaced squats in first-place. I believe that's the result of my greater emphasis on squats – what you focus on grows… especially in your mind.

- Cleans. There are two type of cleans – power cleans and hanging cleans. The first type of clean I learned and used was hanging cleans. They proved to be more effective than power cleans for myself and my teams. After mastering hanging cleans, I progressed to power cleans. I learned both cleans with a pliable object (flour bag) ***before*** cleaning a solid object (bar). That sequence worked best, solidifying my form and building a base of strength. The fundamental differences between hanging cleans and power cleans is the starting point. Power cleans start with the weight on the floor instead of off the floor. The starting point of hanging cleans is the finish line of deadlifts – hanging cleans start with the weight off the floor, standing upright with feet planted on the floor. Both cleans have the same finish line – shoulder level. How the weight gets there is the difference. Power cleans use one complicated motion to get to the finish line – a trap-assisted deadlift with a clean combined with a squat. Hang cleans use two motions – unassisted deadlift to the off-floor starting point, followed by a clean combined with a squat.

My personal preference is hanging cleans for four reasons:

- Hip roll. In addition to the traditional technique, I incorporated a hip roll, a movement that is the difference between becoming a viscous tackler and a tackling dummy. The hip roll is a violent forward thrust of power generated by transferring energy across a short distance at high-speed. The key is the starting point – ass low, arch the lower back, don't slouch, and bend the knees at 45 degrees (exactly like a two-point stance). Then, hold the bar steady, and ***eXplode*** – roll the hips and clean the bar to shoulder level. Forty-five degree knee bend is the key. It's the mid-point of a squat. The thighs are at peak tension. This stance makes you unmovable. And holding the bar, preparing to hang clean builds the mid-point of the squat, the critical break-point of a squat's positive lifting stage. Two-for-one deal – the stance of hang cleans builds squat power. When the hip roll becomes second nature, rookies go from point-zero to tackling machines.
- Builds grip and forearm strength. Holding a heavy weight off the floor is a separate exercise itself. Take advantage of any opportunity to hold heavy weight. Never underestimate the strength-building powers of simply holding a heavy weight. Additionally, hanging cleans are the equivalent of assisted hammer curls. You can overload the stress on forearms with hanging cleans.
- Builds similar leg power as power cleans. Both types of cleans build leg power. I prefer hanging cleans because my two-point stance trains squat lockout, referring to the top half of the squat's positive stage.
- Simpler. The power clean undoubtedly can build power but it's not a simple exercise to master. Both cleans are connected to deadlifts. Power cleans incorporate deadlifts. Hanging cleans separate deadlifts. That makes power cleans more complicated. Hanging cleans are a

simpler skill. With hanging cleans, I use one of two strategies:

» one deadlfit per set at the beginning of the set, or
» one deadlift before each rep.

- Bag carrying. This is a miracle fat-burner. No exercise I have ever done has burned more fat at warp-speed, built a stronger core and strength endurance than carrying a 140-lb burlap bag on my shoulder and slamming it into a pile. The ultimate transformation where fat melts and armour forges, physically and mentally, simultaneously. And no exercise was simpler.

  Three workers per car had to stack 600 burlap bags in six fifty-foot train boxcars, per day. Bags would make a long journey from a packing room to a warehouse, travel on a conveyor belt down an oiled chute to make the bag go from zero-to-sixty in the blink of an eye before landing on a wooden horse in the middle of the box car.. No exercise better develops grip strength than stopping a high-speed bag from splattering on the floor. Crime prevention. A splattered bag was a serious organizational violation. Time and bags are money. Each worker took turns putting a bag onto his shoulder and walking (running) about eight yards to throw the bag onto a pile. Sixteen yards per toss – one weighted, one at body weight… 1,200 reps per day. Not per week or month or year – per day. Rest time was about 30 seconds. No texting, no socializing, no gadget-playing, no self-admiration in mirrors, no changing channels on the TV, no reading muscle magazines between sets. No breaks for protein shakes. No primal screaming, just shut up and work.

Bag carrying has 7 benefits:

- Partial lunge. Every step you take is a weighted partial lunge. A series of partial contraction and tension that builds incredible leg strength.
- Increased stride length X stride frequency. Builds faster speed. Lowers 40-time. 40-yard sprint time is one of the sacred litmus tests used by football recruiters to determine who goes to the next level and who doesn't.
- Core strength. Stabilizing the upper body to support heavy weight armourizes the core.
- Sledgehammer effect. Throwing down a 140-lb bag has the exact same effect as the fashionable sledgehammer training. The repeated upper body tension builds ab-armour better than any ab exercise or ab machine.
- Calorie burning. Calories don't get burned, they get incinerated. You become a calorie-burning furnace physically and mentally. Guaranteed to light your soul on fire. Guaranteed to purge fat-building toxins in the mind and body.
- Cardio-plus. Contrary to popular belief, HIIT (high-intensity interval training) is not a recent invention by the fitness industry. Floor-mill workers benefited from the miracle of wind sprints long before personal trainers did. Intervals of weighted wind sprints and jogging are the best cardiovascular exercise – no exceptions.
- Iron will. Iron-will doesn't just happen. Iron-will is the product of not giving in to imagined exhaustion, referring to the early stage of discomfort that gets magnified by a soft mind. Iron-will is a negative turned into a positive – not quitting when a job gets tough and sticking it out when no one else wants to or can. Finishing a job.

No job I've done has made a bigger impact on my mind, body and soul. Sustained workload, in isolation, no audience, no escape, no excuses. ***Bag carrying knocks the punk out of you.*** When you think you're a tough motherfucker, test your hypotheses with Boxcar Therapy. Carry something heavy for 8 hours with only two choices – get fired up or get fired. It worked on me. It knocked out the punk. Bag carrying has been a staple in my football practices and always will be because of the ***punk-busting effect.*** Bag carrying has been the harshest Darwinian process I have witnessed and experienced. It cuts with the sharpest blade. It has forged my no-cut team philosophy – I never cut players from a football team or from my workouts. They cut themselves when they can't cut the hard work. The secret is to make the training Darwinian in nature – make the struggle tough enough where the weak can't progress…where the weak have to exercise free will to quit or get better. No job has raised my level of consciousness higher more than rep after endless reps of bag carrying. What I learned cannot be taught in any school, from any self-help book or DVD, or from any self-proclaimed motivational speaker.

Squat & press. No exercise developed my core and functional leg strength better than squat & press. I didn't learn this exercise in the gym. I learned it in the same place – boxcar. Squat & press was the only way to reach higher. Each row of burlap bags was higher than my 5'10" height. To reach the top rows, I had to use a simple technique:

- stand the bag upright on my shoulder,
- support the bag with a hammer-grip by holding the bottom of the bag in a V-shaped palms-in pocket,
- squat down to 90 degrees, and
- squat up and press up simultaneously.

Squat & Press is a full-body exercise. There isn't a fiber of body, mind, and soul that doesn't get pumped. Guaranteed to flip the switch. Guaranteed to call out the beast.

These four are the heart and soul of MUSCLE ACADEMY, my pre-season on-field workouts that test balls-size… if they are over-inflated, under-inflated, or up to standard. MUSCLE ACADEMY is my mission statement: ***if you fear hard work, you will not cut it here.*** Muscle Academy is my communications director. It sends out my message: ***Natural talent is not to be feared. Only the beast needs to be feared.*** The beast is the monster that works the hardest. The only fear we have is a team that has out-lifted, outworked or out-trained us. And that won't happen – guaranteed. If it ever does, we will not field a team. I won't be a part of enabling the laziness, entitlement, and insufferable selfish attitudes that disrespect a high-risk sport that can kill or maim. Muscle Academy is Exhibit A that proves my zero tolerance for the plague that risks team safety – laziness. No work ethic. Tolerating laziness is the height of misleadership, the type of leadership that endangers every player and guarantees a culture of losing.

Triangle

In 1985, I added the **Triangle – Hack Squats, Leg Extensions, Leg Curls** – 3 supplementary exercises that serve two purposes:

- Add challenging workload as pre-squat or post-squat fatigue-boosters in supersets or megasets
- An alternative to a day off.

I tried every leg press – 90-degree, 75-degree, 45-degree. In 1990, I eliminated all leg presses because I couldn't get rid of the Lazy-Boy feeling. Leg extensions and leg curls are the only exercises I've kept that don't keep me grounded. Leg exercises are supposed to have both feet planted on the ground. Leg extensions and leg curls are alternatives for a day off and they add workload challenge for squat supersets or megasets. But leg presses have never worked for me or my players. Leg presses are rep-robbers – they represent reps that take away from developing REPxpertise in what matters – building the base.

SHOULDERS-TRAPS-NECK (Tripod)

- Standing Military / Overhead Press
- Seated Military Press
- Hammer Strength Seated Military Press
- DB Hammer Grip Overhead Press
- DB Side Laterals
- Upright rows and shrugs
- Shrugs
- 4-Way Neck Lifts

Allowing any child or adolescent to play any violent, contact sport without developing the TRIPOD is an act of gross negligence. Exposing young girls and boys to the brain-rattling impact without developing shoulders, traps, and neck is the equivalent of any other endangerment… any other safety risk that children are legally protected from.

Editorial #8

When I think of the brain-rattling impact of contact sports, I wonder why any parent would risk their child's brain and spinal cord for the sake of a sport that allows head shots. Hockey is a perfect example of madness, where punching each other in the head is a celebrated by simple-minded coaches, players, and fans who are foolish to believe that toughness is equated to having a controlled 30 second fist-fight. The only reason that hockey players fight is they know someone will stop it – soon. If the referee sent them into a dark alley to fight in isolation, with no audience and no one to break it up, the fighting would stop immediately. Guaranteed. Coaches who send players to fist-fight should be banned from sports. Players who instigate fights by punching another humans head should be banned from sports. In real-life, punching people in the head is a crime. So is counseling it. Celebrating, embracing, and advocating an act that can cause the deadly long-term side-effects from concussion is either a symptom of low-IQ, mental illness, or a criminal mind. There's enough legal violence in contact sports. Illegally punching the opponent in the head is an overt sign of cowardice and incompetence – hardcore evidence that the pugilist is unwilling or incapable of using the legal force that the game allows.

Tripod

I have pushed myself and my players mercilessly through every type of overhead press, shrugs, upright rows, and 4-way neck lifts to build the strongest tripod. As explained in Part 1, the best overhead press is standing Military presses with an Olympic bar. Alternatives are:

- standing Smith machine Military presses,
- seated Olympic bar Military press machine, or
- seated Hammer Strength.

Despite my preference for being grounded as much as possible, the seated Hammer Strength has opened my eyes…and shoulders. Hammer Strength has built my shoulders better than any other exercise, especially when I keep my feet off the ground. Bigger, stronger, more defined. Another example of how an investigation can challenge assumptions with solid evidence.

I never do heavy shrugs in isolation. They are always connected to Military Press or Bench Press to form a higher workload superset or megaset. Shrugs are my alternative to rest between sets. The only way to do shrugs is the simplest – straight up and down. I see people rotating their shoulders doing shrugs and question what goes through their minds. Straight up, straight down. Upright rows finished with a shrug builds enormous tripod mass. After using an Olympic bar for decades, I've switch to cables and a straight bar. The key is the track. Hand placement is essential. Thumbs must align with the outer shoulder. Stay on track until the traps reach maximum contraction. Then lower the bar in slow motion. Don't let the bar free-fall. The negative stage of any lift either builds power or is wasted depending on the speed and control of the weight.

I always superset dumbbell side laterals with dumbbell upright rows/shrugs. I consider it one exercise – no rest, seamless pathway. The combined effect changes the exercises from isolated finishing exercises to a quasi-compound exercise that builds shredded size. I have eliminated bent-over flies for two reasons:

- the combined effect of Hammer strength, dumbbell side laterals, and DB upright rows/shrugs build the back of shoulders better than bent-over flies; and
- rep-conserving. In 1994, I changed my attitude about the time I invest working out. Working out is a significant part of my life but it is not my whole life. Not even close. Working out is part of everyday like eating and breathing but working out does not consume me. I have a many other professional and personal interests far outside working out. I became a better investor and conservationist. ***I learned to invest less with much higher returns. I learned to conserve time with better energy.*** What's important is not the quantity of the investment – quality matters more that quantity. I cut down down-time and redundant exercises. I did an exercise inventory. Bent-over DB flies were the first to get cut. As more exercises got cut, so did I.

Neck lifts are simple. Lay on a flat bench, hold a weight on your forehead, and lift up with your neck to only 45-degrees. Lower your head to the starting point only – flat. No lower. My starting point is a parallel head, to force the neck to remain tense while holding the weight. The movement should look like an ab crunch using the head. The same movement applies to the side and the back – don't lower the weight father that parallel. Keep maximum tension.

BACK

- Chins - underhand
- Chins - overhand
- BB Bent-Over Rows (T-bar & bags)
- DB single-arm rows
- Cable Pulldowns - underhand
- Cable Pulldowns - overhand

V-shape will not happen unless you cut fat off your belly and call for **back-up**. I did only three back exercises for my first six years – underhand chins (close), overhand chins (wide), and bent-over rows with bags ranging from 100-140 lbs.

Close grip chins build up arms and blow up the back. Two-for-one deal. I used to question why I included underhand chins as a back exercise because I got a bigger arm pump than a back pump. Then I realized that chins were a back-up exercise – use your back to get up first, then call your biceps for back-up. I was using arms for the first 2-inch explosion for three years until re-focused. I consciously started using my lats for the 2-inch explosion. Order was restored. Back blew up first and my arms became the back-up. Change the focus, change the outcome.

The problem with underhand chins is they get too easy because of biceps back-up. You need a weighted belt or superset or focus more on wide-grip overhand chins or all of the above. Wide-grip overhand chins don't get easy because there's no arm back-up.

Chins are not easy to learn. If you can't do a chin-up, do floor chins… the equivalent of training wheels for chin-ups. Real chin-ups need a bar overhead, a vertical lift with strict vertical body position, and feet off the floor. Floor chins have both feet on the floor, the torso at 45-degrees, and the bar at chest height.

Bent-over rows with a bag took over first place as a V-shaper. Holding a bag requires a hammer-grip – palms-in, facing each other. Huge difference from holding an Olympic bar. My alternative now is a T-bar row that replicates the bag grip. Bent-over rows accomplish the same as deadlifts – the weight is lifted off the ground for approximately the same distance. The difference is the torso position – upright torso versus bent-over torso. The key to bent-over rows is to not bend-over at 90 degrees. The best results have been achieved at a torso angle of 45 degrees forward. This angle focuses the attention on the back. Using an open-grip (thumb off the handle instead of around it) increases the focus on the lats and away from arms. But, it's impossible to cancel arms as back-up. Back and arms are connected.

I still use single-arms bent-over DB rows but they do not produce the same results as two-arm rows. The reason is that any one-arm-at-a-time exercise does not generate the full-pump as does using both arms. Personally, I don't like the half-pump feeling. And it needlessly extends my gym time. One-arm exercises double the amount of time needed to accomplish the same results as two-arm. Contrary to myth, one-arm rows do not produce any different results than two-arm rows. Believing that they are different is a casualty of conformity – we believe what we want to believe and disregard the rest.[14]

As my equipment grew, so did my alternatives. I added cable pulldowns (underhand and over hand) and seated cable rows. There are three directions of rows. Each one has a relationship with gravity:

- upward through gravity, i.e., bent-over rows
- across gravity, i.e., seated rows
- with gravity, i.e., pulldowns.

The positive stage of pulldowns is gravity-assisted, the negative stage is not. Pulldowns help develop chin power by replicating the chin movement backwards – chins bring the body to the bar, pulldowns bring the bar to the body. I use pulldowns for supersets and alternative to rest days. Done properly, pulldowns will build back mass. I've watched in horror as lifters wildly heave and swing and bounce and throw themselves back while doing pulldowns. Like symptoms of impairment – erratic pulldowns. It's a miracle people don't crack their skulls while violently leaning backwards. Pulldowns have a strict stance and track. The best underhand grip aligns the inside of the fists with the outside of the shoulders. I tilt my head back at 30-degrees, aligning my chest under the bar and keeping my back rigid with my shoulder arched back at 15-degrees. My elbows follow a track tight with the ribs. The elbows have to lower as close as possible to the torso – no space between the elbows and the ribs. The bottom of the positive stage is the elbow even with

14 Tribute to a masterpieeece, *The Boxer*. By Simon & Garfunkel. "*A man hears what he wants to hear and disregards the rest.*" Music is a force that drives gym performance. I'll discuss the magic of gym music later in the book but here's what has worked for me – an eclectic Ipod. I used to respond exclusively to the heaviest metal to lift heavy metal. But my music listening has grown exponentially. My workout Ipod includes every type of music imaginable.

the ribs – not before. Then, slow motion during the negative stage to fight gravity. The maniacs who let the weight fly upward and slam the weight stack are risking serious injury as they try to dislodge their shoulders from their sockets while having no regard for gym property. Letting plates smash is a symptom of two problems: weakness of mind, weakness of body, and weakness of character. In other words, laziness and stupidity.

True underhand pulldowns use a straight bar – palms facing your face. But the best pulldown success I've experienced is using any bar that allows for Hammer Grip – palms facing each other other. Hammer grip pulldowns produce more strength and mass than any other true underhand or overhand pulldown.

The key to wide overhand pulldowns is hand placement and track. Everything is the same as underhand. I align thumbs outside the shoulder, same stance as underhand pulldowns and same track – elbows tight to torso.

The best rows are T-bar row with a hammer-grip. The key is stance. I use a football 2-point stance – feet under shoulders, ass low, torso at 45-degrees, chin up. Elbow track is the same as pulldowns – tight against the ribs.

I eliminated seated cable rows ten years ago. The reason was rep-conservation and investment. I experimented with every technique humanly possible and could not find the magical back pump. No matter how hard I tried, I could not eliminate arm back-up during the 2-inch liftoff that starts the positive stage. Seated rows worked my arms more than my back – and I didn't need another arm exercise. When an exercise doesn't produce, I cut it. The exercises that survive are the only ones that yield the highest return for the lowest investment.

∞

Part 4.3.2:
Arms – Triceps, Biceps, Forearms, Grip

Item 1. ARMS are a team. "ARMS" is the unification of 4 forces: biceps, triceps, forearms, and grip. I've tried every type of workout combination – push/pull together and pull & push alone. Biceps and triceps together (push/pull together), biceps alone, triceps alone, biceps & back (pull together), chest triceps (push together). I've concluded that ARMS produces the best results. Nothing else comes close.

Item 2. Biceps are not just beach muscles. They are the foundation for every upper body exercise, every football skill, every law enforcement survival skill, and every labour-intensive job. The first time I heard the *biceps are beach muscles* nonsense, I knew that the fitness industry was capable of complicating, contradicting, and confounding the simplest of basic fundamentals. Imagine ignoring biceps. Imagine a half-developed arm. Simplicity is ignored when simplicity is either not sexy and glamorous or too hard to do.

Item 3. The psychology of arms build-up – *One of the differences between winning and losing is being frightened or frightening.* Even though narcissism may be a sign of a deeper problem, rolling up the jersey sleeves on a football field to show arms build-up is a powerful way to send a message – *we won't be outworked.* No message frightens the competition more. A tireless team is a frightening team. A tireless team is a machine that *WILL NOT QUIT*. A tireless team is a beast that will not give in, will not back down, and will not go away no matter what happens. All of this can be conveyed by simply rolling up the sleeves.

Rolling up the sleeves was evidence of the turning point when my football team went from the nightmare of a winless season in 1984 to a perfect season in 1985. Big arms intimidated the opposition by planting anticipated pain in their minds. No one can think or act at their best when they focus on fear of anticipated pain. The anticipation of pain is worse than the real thing. Words don't frighten. they don't scare anyone except the exceptionally soft-minded and weak-willed. Statements don't carry weight. The best way to send a frightening message to the opposition is non-verbal communication – physical evidence. And nothing grabs attention better than arms build-up. Nothing sends a message better – tireless, blue-collar, won't back down, will mess you up, bust you up, and fuck you up.

Part 4.3.3:
Triceps

TRICEPS
- Dips
- Close-Grip Bench Press
- Close-Grip Pushup
- Cable Pulldowns
- Cable Rope Extensions, aka: Skullcrushers / French Press

Ten years ago, I cut my Sacred Triceps list to these five. I got rid of everything else – kickbacks, machine triceps extensions, and every form of bar/DB triceps extensions (seated or lying) except rope extensions on a cable machine. The reasons are productivity and injury-prevention. The five Sacred Triceps Exercises combined with chest presses build more shredded triceps landmass than you'll ever need. And every triceps extension has eventually lead to tendonitis or some other needless triceps pain. The only exception are lying rope extensions on a cable machine. The reason is the hammer-grip and stability. A cable-machine rope attachment allows only the hammer grip. A straight bar doesn't. Hammer grip prevents tendon tension and isolates fully on the triceps. Although DBs permit hammer grip, the rope attachment provides better stability by ensuring a stable stance and track. The rope locks my elbows at 45-degrees away from my skull and locks my fists onto one consistent track. Pain-free for over a decade.

I use a specially-made dip-bar with fat-handles. Fat-handles blow up triceps. The secret is the wide open-grip – the thumb and finger don't touch – there's a 3-inch space that separates them. A fat-grip dip-bar prevents a closed-grip, and recruits more triceps fibers, calling out the full force of the triceps. I never go lower that 90-degree arm angle because 90-degrees forces the triceps (instead of elbow tendons and ligaments) to support bodyweight. This is the key to preventing mangling tendons and ligaments – force the muscle to support the weight during the positive-negative transition. I apply this to every exercise, every bodypart. Bodyweight dips are an essential power source.

F.A.Q.s:

What's a respectable number of bodyweight reps?

Minimum of 19. That's the threshold forcing you to cross into the 20's.

How do you know when it's time to progress to weighted dips?

Same answer as above.

What's the reps goal for weighted dips?

1RM doesn't apply to weighted dips.

Most rookies I've coached have trouble doing one dip. What's the best strategy to do one full dip when you can't do even partial dips.

Keep extending the distance dipped until you reach one full rep.

What's the secret to improving reps after you get the first one?

- Straight-line power. Stability. Stop swinging erratically. Zero momentum – stop at the bottom briefly…find the sweet spot where the triceps are doing all the work. ***eXplode*** on liftoff, lockout will follow – guaranteed.
- Occasionally, I have replaced close-grip bench press for a few weeks just to change things up. The only change that happened was triceps size and strength. Power outage – weakness. There are direct relationships between close-grip bench and:
    - » 225RM bench press
    - » 1RM bench press
- Winning and losing because of striking power, referring to any skill (and sport) that requires explosive arm extension.
- There is no such thing as doing close-grip bench press for too long. You can do them every triceps day. They never go stale.
- Close-grip pushups are connectors – I almost always connect them to another exercise to form a superset or megaset. I use several hand placements:
    - » full triangle – index fingers and thumbs touching
    - » open triangle – index fingers and thumbs separated by 2 inches
    - » rectangle – thumbs touching, index fingers open facing vertically
    - » open rectangle – hands under shoulders
- Use full-range slow motion. Chest touches back of hands, contract at top, full control, no wild up-down piston-action.
- Pushdowns with Fat Gripz on a V-shape short bar are triceps-blasters. How you do them determines whether you build triceps mass or waste your time. Pushdowns are the opposite of barbell curls – same stance, same track, opposite direction. Pushdown positives are down, instead of up for curls. The 2 keys are :
    - » **Stance**: open-grip (thumb on top), elbows hinged at the front of the torso, not the back.
    - » **Track**: lock the elbows. Elbows act as a stationary hinge. Full range. Slow motion. Stop at the bottom, stop at the top. Torso vertically rigid.
- Pushdown derivatives include a forward stance – lean forward at 45 degrees, elbows hinged and locked away from torso, fists near forehead. Push toward bottom of the weight stack, form a 45-degree track from forehead to the stack.

Part 4.3.4:
Biceps – Forearms

BICEPS – Forearms
- BB Curls
- DB 1-Arm Curls
- Cable EZ Curls - standing
- Hammer Bar Cable Curls

BICEPS – 4 F-Bombs
- Hammer Curls
- V-Hammer Curls
- Reverse Curls
- Wrist Rolls - Standing BB, Standing DB, Standing Cable

Bend your arm at 90-degrees. Made a fist and flex your arm. Look at the V-shape formed by the forearm and side of the upper arm. It's a **shield**. Now, imagine someone running at you, trying to knock you on your ass. Lift your arm outward towards the hostile... ***strike the shield.*** That's my basic football security skill that I teach for any position – for blockers who have to move tacklers, for tacklers who have to shed blockers, for ball-carriers who have to shed tacklers. The shield is not just self-defense – it's self-*offense*.

Now, imagine you're a cop at a 911 call. Or a domestic dispute. Or a bar disturbance. Some place where minds under substance-influence are causing social havoc. Now, imagine a bad guy trying to throw a punch at your head or ribs... any place above the waist. Lift your shield like an uppercut so that your fist is at the side of your skull. The V-shape shield is protecting you head, face, and torso. That's one of the basic survival skills that I have taught college wannabe cops.

I'm not a self-defense instructor and never have been. I'm a survival coach. I teach book smarts and street smarts to get a job done while staying in one piece. Intellectual training is just as important as physical training. My job is to prevent my student-athletes from getting busted up.

Why are biceps and forearms important? To build three things – the shield, the weapons and the lifting machine... the ARMS. Biceps and forearms are the armour and artillery that protect and serve. Every press and pull movement depends on the lifting machine called the "ARMS" to support the weight being pushed and pulled.

Biceps and forearms are connected – inseparable. My Scared Bicep/Forearms Exercises are divided into two groups of four: B-4 (four biceps exercises), 4 F-Bombs (four Forearm Bombs that ***eXplode*** the forearms). Every biceps workout I've done in my life has included standing barbell curls. Every single one. No exception. From my first arm workout, 42 years ago, to last night. Do I get bored of BB curls? No. Do my arms get stale? No. I don't need to confuse my arms, trick them, or subject them to any gimmicks. I need to combine heavy low reps with challenging high reps. I need to feel my biceps bursting. BB curls does the trick every time – guaranteed. The secret to dynamic curls are:

- stance & track – fists to shoulders;
- elbow hinge – lock the elbow into the front half of the torso;
- weight transfer – push down on feet as you *eXplode* the two-inch liftoff;
- slow motion downward;
- don't swing like a drunkard leaving a bar at closing time – stay solid as a statue;
- zero momentum – stop the weight at the bottom and the top; and
- use FAT GRIPZ – your arms will transform.

I always stand, never sit. Standing develops 2-point stance power, balance, and stability. I always use a straight bar for free weight curls, never an EZ-curl bar. I scrapped seated Preacher/ Scott Curls over a decade ago because:

- the front of my elbow felt like it was tearing in half or being stabbed;
- the pump, power, and muscle size never came close to standing curls; and
- sitting is too comfortable.

if you're going to do 3-4 sets of Preacher Curls, just do 3-4 more standing curls. My investigation has found zero evidence that proves seated curls are needed to "hit" the biceps differently. I never did a preacher curl during my first 6 years of working out. I did only standing BB curls and standing DB Hammer curls exclusively during that time. Those two standing exercises were directly responsible for a 300 lb. 1RM bench press, 18 reps at 225, and 18-inch arms before my 18th birthday… naturally. And not one supplement because I never heard of them and couldn't afford them if I had. My only supplement was iron.

Although I fight conformity like an evil enemy, I still release my inner conformist occasionally by adding single-arm DB curls, cable EZ-bar curls, and hammer-bar cable curls, reverse curls, and V-Hammer curls.

If I wanted to simplify my biceps/forearms workout to its rawest form, I would only do the same two exercises I did when I was 12 – standing BB curls and standing DB Hammer curls. These two always have and always will build massive, shredded arms. Nothing else compares. Standing BB curls build the front of the biceps, DB Hammer curls build the forearm (especially the all-important inner forearm that pushes through bench press break points to guarantee lock-out) and the outside of the upper arm… the top part of the shield. DB Hammer curls have the same principles as BB curls except the palms are facing each other while the fist forms a hammer-head. At the end of every Hammer curls set, I do standing wrist rolls holding the DB in front of the torso with arms bent at 90-degrees.

Last night's biceps and forearm workout was a perfect example of how I blasted my arms beyond human comprehension at the age of 54. I did only two exercises – standing BB curls and standing DB Hammer curls using a SPLIT DROP-ADD Concept – illustrated below:

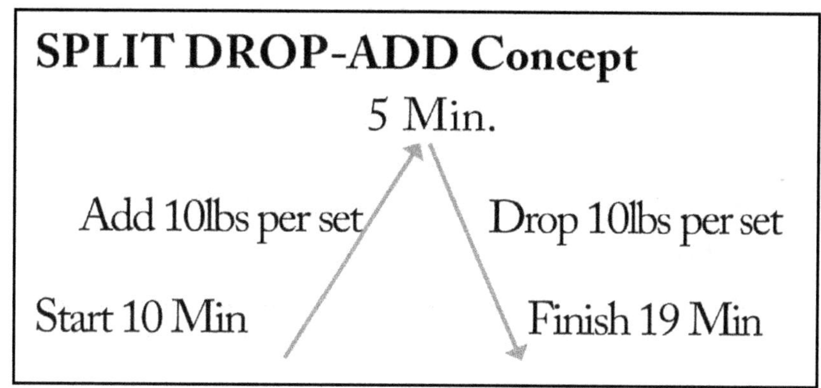

Split DROP-ADD means a Drop-set and Add-set combined but split instead of consecutive. The goal is to start with a weight that allows a minimum of 19 reps using challenging weight so the last 5 reps are heavy enough to represent 5RM heavyweight (through fatigue). Add 10 lbs. on each subsequent set until you reach 5RM. The key is to test every fiber of mental and physical strength. Don't cheat yourself by giving into discomfort and concealing reps. When you reach the 5 rep min., strip the weight…10 lbs. at a time. Climb down the ladder you built on the way up. The rest between sets is 20-reps of abs. No other rest.

Here's what I did last night:

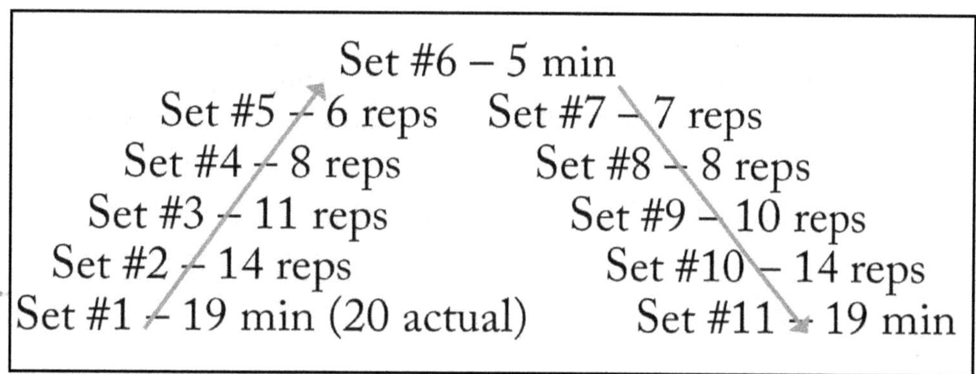

- 6 sets climbing up at 10-lb increments to 5 RM
- 5 sets down stripping 10 lbs. each set (almost the same reps)
- Weight selection: start at 25% BW to 55% BW
- 11 sets total
- 121 reps (biceps)
- 220 reps (abs)
- Total time = est. 20 minutes
- I followed with a 5-set SPLIT DROP-ADD for DB Hammer Curls:

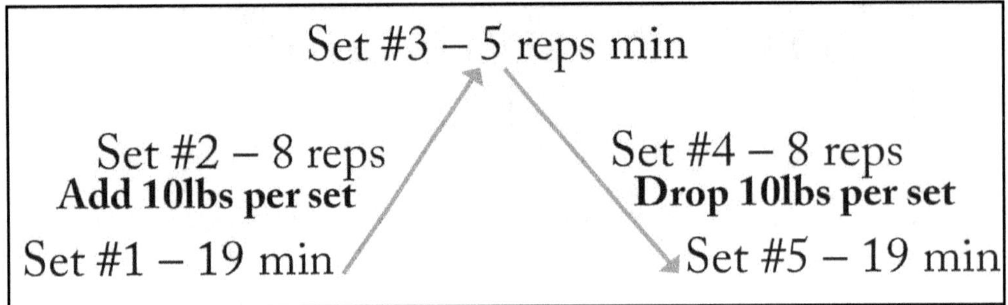

- Supersetted with standing wrist rolls (the only rest period)
- 59 reps Hammer Curls
- 59 reps wrist rolls
- 119 total reps

The total reps for the full workout was 239.

Total sets = 32.

Total time = 30 minutes.

Result = massive arms build-up.

- **DB 1-arm curls** have a purpose – isolated pressure by single-arm stress. The curling capacity of one arm is not half or double the capacity for 2 arms curling simultaneously. You'll curl less than half the weight of 2-arm curls. Curling with one arm at a time exerts isolated pressure, making it harder to curl than with 2 arms.
- **Standing Cable EZ-bar curls** have 3 benefits over straight-bar free weight curls:

  i. Greater positive & negative resistance. Good cables make the positive heavier and the negative faster, forcing a greater use of force.

  ii. The 45-degree upward hand position on the EZ bar is a 50% hammer-grip, providing a 50-50 split focus on bicep and forearm.

  iii. Great alternative when the gym is busy and the Olympic bars are taken.

- **Hammer-bar** cable changes the 50-50 focus to 75-25 in favour of forearms, building incredible forearms and top shield (the outer upper arm). A hammer-bar is a straight bar with vertical handles on the end that position the palms facing in, with fists moving up and down like a hammer.
- **V-Hammer curls** have the opposite effect of EZ-bar, using a downward 45-degree stance and track that splits the focus – a 50-50 forearm/biceps ratio. Hold the DB with downward 45-degree grips, bars against the hips. Lift at 45-degrees, touch the DB at the chest. The track of the DBs is 45 degrees upward to the chest, instead of the vertical 90-degrees hammer curl track to the shoulders. The 45-degree track forms an inverted V.
- **Reverse curls** are awkward if you use a full closed grip on a straight bar. I never use a full grip for straight-bar reverse curls. Instead, I use a partial 60% grip, using the thumb, index finger,

and middle finger only. The fourth and fifth fingers are off the bar. The reason is to increase isolated pressure on the inside of the forearms. Alternatives are reverse EZ curls with a bar or DB. The downward 45-degree grips and vertical upward track to the shoulders provides a 50-50 split focus.

- All other **bicep exercises** got cut from my Sacred Exercises list. Overhead curls standing between 2 weight stacks… cut. Seated isolated DB curls with elbows locked against the knee – cut. Using an arm blaster to lock the elbows – cut. I learned that locking the elbow into a proper hinge position without the use of a stationary object increases the difficulty by increasing the workload, increasing the isolated pressure, and increasing the discipline of doing something the strict, correct way using your own power, your own energy source. More challenging, more muscle – mentally and physically.

Part 4.3.5:
ABs

I've learned four rules of ab-cutting:

Rule #1: The only ab-magic is fat – fat makes abs disappear.
Abs are like the weather – clear or cloudy. There's a blurry line separating visible from invisible abs. That line is made up of fat. Fat is cloud cover.... abs-blockers. Making fat disappear needs more than magic. It needs a combination of hard work, consistent self-discipline, iron-will, and keeping your mouth shut to regulate access of junk.

Rule #2: Six-packs obscure six packs. There's no magic exercise that, by itself, will give you a visible six-pack. No exercise, no machine, no magic pill beats a junk diet. If you are a human garburator, nothing will cut the fat or cut your abs.

Rule #3: The magic fat-burner – lift iron, stop lifting junk food, and lift your feet. Lifting souls, lifting soles – the proactive approach that prevents the three leading causes of fat build-up... iron deficiency, protein deficiency, and cardio deficiency.

Rule #4: If you don't spill your guts, your gut will spill over. Getting fat is easy. It took me less than a year of inactivity, as a child, laid-up in a leg cast to become obese. Losing fat is not easy. Fat loss doesn't just happen. Keeping it off doesn't just happen. You have to spill your guts to lose your gut.

Rule #5: Waste mismanagement leads to waist mismanagement. It's impossible to discuss abs without talking about food, iron, and running. There is a direct relationship between a flat stomach and resistance training, eating, and cardio. Abs are the scoreboard for the fat-fighting battle. Love handles and paunches are the result of mismanagement – waste mismanagement that leads to waist mismanagement. Eliminate the waste to reduce the waist.

I am a fat loss expert... a professional fat-fighter. I have fought fat for over four decades, I am not a genetically-gifted lean-machine athlete, I have no natural talent, but I was built naturally – no fat-burners, no surgeries, no needles, no steroids, no performance-enhancing drugs. And no nutritionists, no coaches. Guided by the Soul of a Lifter. Self-educated. Voracious reading and real-life experimenting. Here's how I cleared up the issue of abs... my fat loss plan:

- Carb-regulation. I am a purebred Italian which means I'm pureBREAD addicted. I grew up on carbs for two reasons: i) my parents came from Italy, penniless – carbs were all they could afford, and ii) carbs fuel manual labour. Blue-collar workers don't give a shit about carb-cutting. During my first 2 decades of working out, carbs were my natural anabolic agent. Carbs gave me unnatural power, strength and size. That feeling can get you hooked on even more carbs. Then, when the bulk gets too much, I cut-up by cutting carbs until I feel like I'm weakening and resort to carb-inhalation. Viscous cycle of carb-regulation and carb-inhalation.

- Striking the carb-balance has been a life-long battle. The perfect carb-balance scores three points – clear abs + vascularity + mass + a full tank. Perfect carb-balance gives you a lean waist without losing shredded size and without the energy depletion that accompanies card-reduction. The bad news about striking the carb-balance is this – having fought the fat-battle without chemical re-engineering, pharmaceuticals, and anabolic agents, I don't strike the perfect balance often. Something gets sacrificed. If my abs clear up, I'm running on fumes and my clothes get baggy. If my tank is full, my abs get cloudy. To clear up abs, I cut out bread and pasta. The only way that I come close to striking the balance is using a 10-point plan that features a protein-packed, carb-regulated diet – same meals every day. Same food routine. REPS – repeatedly eating protein systemically. Eating the same meals has been life-altering. It's made long-term impact. It's not a gimmick, it's a life-style.

- 10-point plan. I'm stronger and leaner at 54 than when I was 24. The following 10-point plan is my anti-aging secret:

i. Six protein intakes daily. Protein every 2-3 hours is essential to maintain positive nitrogen balance. Translation – a steady stream of protein makes you strong and hard 24/7. My six meals are more like a seamless path of food during waking hours. The secret is portion-size and protein-size. Never get full and 30 grams of protein per intake. I have 4 protein sources: egg whites, fish, chicken, whey protein. That's it. I stay away from red meat.

ii. Carbs during the first half of the day, zero carbs during the second half of the day. My carb sources are sweet potatoes, brown rice, spinach, broccoli, and brussel sprouts. That's it.

iii. 2 litres of water mixed with BCAA (Branch Chain Amino Acids). I carry the 2 litres jug everywhere. I drink it over 16 hours.

iv. I run 45 minutes almost every day of my life – at least 26 out of 28 days. Every other day, I include wind sprints at the end of the run.

v. I don't have one cheat day. I have several. My workouts are brutally intense every day. I run out of gas easily. When I feel like shit, I carb-up – including the carbs I'm not supposed to eat. Pizza, bagels, roasted potatoes just to mention a few. Life is too short to be carb-deprived every day of your life. Being carb-deprived is painful. When I'm running low, I can't think straight. My head gets fuzzy. I start stuttering, some slurred speech, bloodshot eyes, edgy, unruly, disagreeable – like a drunk. As soon as I feel the onset of carb-deprivation, the switch turns on. Carb-inhalation. I never have and never will count calories or grams of carbs or grams of fat or grams of protein. The reason is evidence. I have paid attention to what works for me and what doesn't. I know what I need to eat, when, and exactly how much. Evidence takes time to find but any discovery needs work.

vi. Zero fast food. I recognized a long time ago that I don't have an off-switch.

vii. Zero alcohol. I recognized a long time ago that I don't have an off-switch. The only bars I've been in during my adult life are the ones I was required to attend as a police office to break up fights, arrest knife attackers, women-beaters, and other public safety threats.

viii. Iron. I lift intensely. I force my body to work in overdrive and overtime. The real reason for the intensity is the H-bomb – hormone bombs. It flips the testosterone and growth hormone switch. Free, legal, and 100% natural. Don't let the H-bombs drop. Testosterone starts free-falling at thirty-something unless you turn on the switch regularly. Once testosterone dips to drips, you'll be asked for ID, long before becoming a senior, to get your 15% discount. You'll replace cutoffs with cardigans before you reach forty. Intense workouts open a window of growth opportunity. There's a 20-60 minute opportunity after each intense workout to get lean and mean simply by consuming protein and carbs (as soon as possible after the workout, within one hour of the last rep).

ix. 8 hours of sleep. Less than that, I get fat.

x. Leave a poisoned workplace. I changed careers when my workplace flipped the wrong switch – the deadly cortisol switch. Cortisol has many nicknames – fight or flight hormone, fat hormone, aging hormone, death hormone. Cortisol is a paradox – it has a good side and a bad side. Getting pissed off flips the cortisol switch. Stress unleashes a torrent of cortisol in your body to prepare it for a physical fight. Cortisol has to be used up immediately with physical exertion. If you don't and simply go back to your cruiser or classroom or cubicle, fat builds-up...physically and mentally. Unused cortisol clouds over your abs. I found a true ab-magic solution – self-employment. I left behind two got-it-made jobs and started my own business. Then another one. My body-fat dropped to single-digits. There's the secret to cutting your abs – be your own boss. My abs were not connected only to Sacred Exercises. My abs were not connected only to carb-regulation. Defined abs are also connected to self-truth. A lengthy self-investigation solved the self-deception that was flooding cortisol and causing a natural disaster. Soul-searching raised my level of consciousness. Here's what I discovered:

- I am not cut out to work for other people. A para-military rank organization was great was I was 18. It was great for awhile while I needed it...until my eyes opened.
- I despise having my life, my destiny, and my potential controlled by strangers.
- I am an ultra non-conformist, extremely unconventional, and I think too far outside the box – an obvious mismatch for public sector administrators. I'll never be in-place trying to fit in at an organization whose ideologies are a total mismatch to mine. Philosophical differences don't get ironed out. The situation just gets worse. Being out-of-place throws off the alignment. Mind, body, and soul get off-track.
- I am easily susceptible to boredom. I suffer deeply from the monotony of sameness. When a job becomes unchallenging and I can't control raising the bar, clouds roll in and darkness sets in.
- Gossiping, back-stabbing, juvenile workplaces poison mind, body, and soul.
- Personal missions change. We have several callings, not just one. Ignoring a new calling is hell.

Becoming a full-time business owner, a full-time writer, a full-time coach, and full-time professional athlete has been a consciousness-lifting, body-fat reducing, six-pack transformation – physically and mentally. It's almost impossible to get your body-fat to single digits naturally while working on someone else's schedule. Example - shift work. Fifteen years of an absurd, barbaric police shift work schedule single-handedly destroyed my inner clock. You can't decline a 911 call on the grounds that you need a protein shake. You can't go home in the middle of a last-minute investigation because you need to recover from a leg workout. You can't fail to appear in court at 10 a.m. after finishing a shift 3 hours earlier because you have a titanic arm workout scheduled. Like any destructive behaviour that you're in the throes of, you can't see how it's fucking you up because heightened awareness takes longer to develop than 18-inch natural arms.

- Iron-will. Mindset is the most important ab-development, fat loss factor. None of the above matters without the self-discipline to make it happen. Self-discipline isn't strong enough, not the word and not the concept. Iron-will is the only solution to fighting fat and cutting abs. Those who can't cut it blame the gym, the coach, the program, everything but their own will. Fat loss and cut abs are the product of free-will exercise – decisions. Choices. It's simple to know how to eat right. It's not quantum physics to know what is not right to eat and drink. What's junk is not a secret, it's not a mystery. Nutrition IQ is largely selective knowledge – wo/man hears what they want to hear and disregards the rest.[15]

They call it "getting wasted" for a reason. Calories from alcohol consumption are a waste. I have warned players thousands of times – there is a direct correlation between getting wasted and losing – losing muscle, losing money, losing brain cells, losing games, and not losing fat. There's a steep price for a brief escape from reality. And when you return, it's the same old place[16]...except worse. As a rookie head coach, I took losing personally. Every loss prompted deep soul-searching, intense self-investigation...until informants told me the truth – the obvious that I had chosen to ignore. Certain players were getting wasted the night before a game. The enemy wasn't my play-calling or my playbook or my coaching or my philosophy or my ideology. Debauchery debilitates. No level of coaching beats a hangover. I wasn't their parent or their legal guardian. I was a part of their lives – the loudspeaker of their conscience. If my voice got shouted down by the voices of their inner demons, it technically wasn't my fault for losing the battle. To my defence, free will was still under the exclusive ownership of each player. I could't be with them 24/7 to fight their battles with forces of evil. I coached them in the gym (if they did't fail to appear) and on the field (if they did't fail to appear). We all have 8,760 hours every year. Equal clock time. What we do with it is the product of fitness – free-will exercise. My actual physical coaching presence with players represents only 2% of their lives. That's not an even playing field compared to their other influences.

- 5-step AB-ladder. After decades of experimenting with every ab exercise known to wo/man-kind, I have selected the five Sacred Ab Exercises – the 5-step ab-ladder:

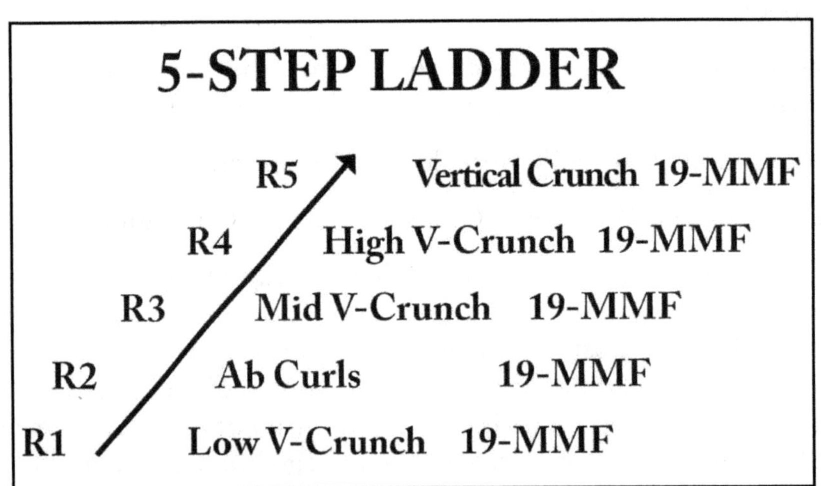

Frequency, volume, and positioning of ab work depends on **Set-Calling©** decisions. How often, how many sets and reps, and where abs fit in the workout are the product of what happened

15 Second tribute to the masterpiece, *The Boxer*. By Simon & Garfunkel.

16 Tribute to a masterpiece, *Eve of Destruction*. Written by P. F. Sloan. Made famous by singer Barry McGuire

in the past and what I'm trying to accomplish at the moment. The two primary factors are two types of recovery:

i. Ab-recovery. Soreness vs tightness. Two separate feelings. Soreness is a red light – don't do them. Abs need recovery. Tight abs is a green light – do them. They have recovered enough and are in the armour-building stage.

ii. Super-set recovery. To reduce down time and still let other bodyparts recover.

The 5-step AB-ladder works for me. It has transformed my abs into my fifties.

Conclusion

What's the secret to never quitting working out? **Athletic Mindset.** Be an athlete. That's the secret. Everyone who regularly exercises is an athlete. Call yourself an athlete and you'll workout forever. Change your perspective of working out – it's a career, not a hobby, not a pain in the ass. Focus on the rush – the rush of the challenge, the rush of being different, the rush of achieving the unachievable, the rush of lifting something heavy, the rush of running on pavement, the rush of H-bombs and the resulting physical pump, intellectual pump, emotional pump, and spiritual pump.

See the beauty and strength of which your body is capable.

Enjoy the book?

We would like to hear from you.

Post a review on Amazon, Goodreads or let us know directly at reviews@ginoarcaro.com.

Follow Gino & Jordan Publications Inc. on Social Media

GinoArcaro *or* GinoArcarco.Author

@Gino_Arcaro *or* @JordanPubInc.

+GinoArcaro *or* +GinoArcaroBooks

GinoArcaro

Gino's Blog

More Books by Gino Arcaro

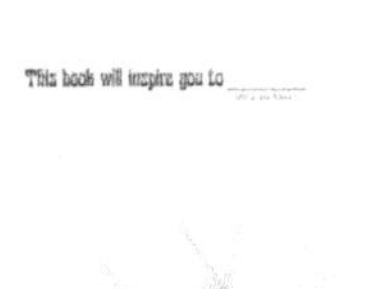

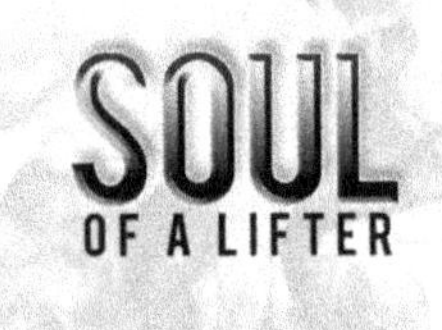

SOUL OF A LIFTER

Gino Arcaro's journey from childhood obesity to natural health and strength was not made alone; he relied on the Soul of a Lifter. In telling this tale, Arcaro draws on life lessons learned from his careers as a football coach, police officer and college teacher to inspire and lead the reader in a soul-searching quest to reach his/her own potential. This is not your run-of-the-mill motivational book. Discover insights about what drives the soul… what happens when you listen and when you don't!

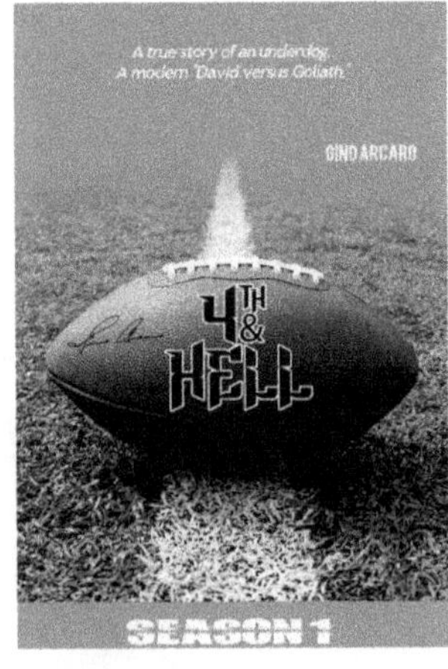

4TH & HELL SEASON 1

"We were David with a Canadian passport, failing miserably at winning just one football game against stars-and-stripes-draped Goliaths." It came down to fourth and hell – a face-to-face showdown. No disguises, no masks, no secret weapons. No one huddled on the sideline. No one huddled on the field. Both sides knew what to expect. No surprises, no guess-work, no mind games. Making the call was a formality. All that mattered was running the play to see what would pass. Someone would execute; someone would be executed.

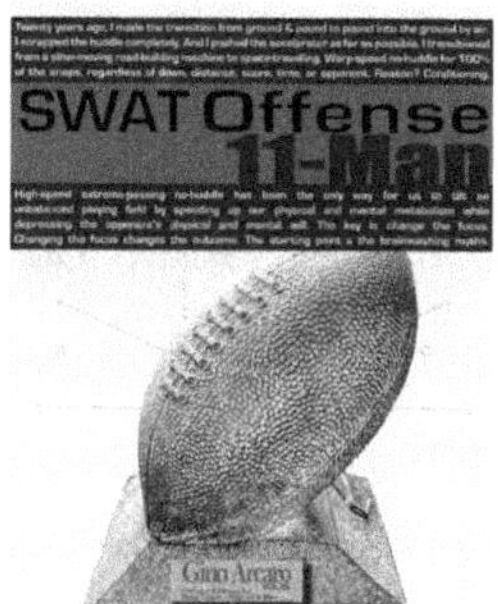

SWAT Offense

By connecting partial concepts that can build any formation, any pass play and any running play to fit the situation, at the line of scrimmage, Arcaro has designed a system that eliminates the need for a conventional playbook that has to be memorized. Memorization is replaced by translation of a simple language. He designed the SWAT offense as a solution to a nightmarish reality of limitations – poor talent and poor resources, a one-man coaching staff, open-admission players, and on top of it all, out-matched opponents willingly sought out! David constantly calling out Goliath. Arcaro's SWAT offense is the most unique offensive system you'll ever see because it has limitless offense capacity but no playbook. A unique feature of the SWAT Offense is its ties to SWAT Defense.

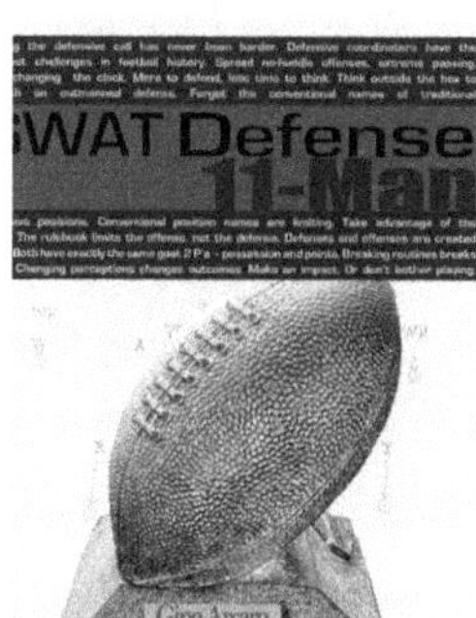

SWAT Defense

Making the defensive call has never been harder. Coordinators have the greatest challenges in football history. Spread no-huddle offenses, extreme passing, clock-changing rules. More to defend, less time to think. Arcaro's SWAT Defense shows how to beat the spread by forcing the offense to go deep and crack under pressure. "A stress-filled workplace for quarterbacks and receivers leads to an explosion." Central to Arcaro's system is his decision-making model that teaches defensive coordinators and players to make the right calls – those split-second decisions that have to be made about 60 times per game. Making the right call is not easy. Like any skill, defensive decision-makers need guidelines and experience to develop into full potential. A unique feature of the SWAT Defense is its ties to Arcaro's SWAT Offense.

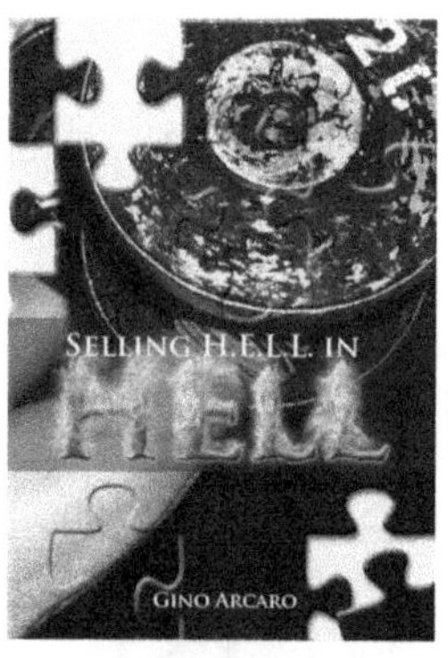

Selling H.E.L.L. in Hell
from the series Soul of an Entrepreneur

You may be starting out in business or just contemplating making the big decision. Gino Arcaro knows what you're thinking and wants to make sure you know what you're not thinking. His thought-bending tales, while entertaining and steeped in reality, will make the would-be business owner take a second and third look at the situation before jumping in. And, for those already "self-employed," Arcaro offers a unique slant on dealing with day-to-day customer and employee challenges.

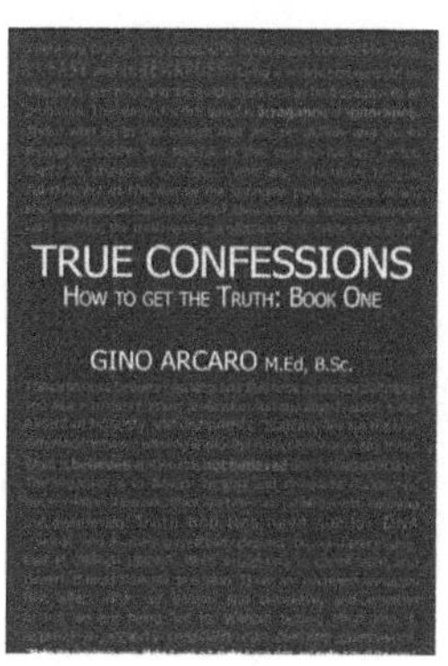

True Confessions

Gino Arcaro relates and upholds a simple fact: "Everyone has a conscience. No exceptions. If you're alive, you have a conscience. The myth of 'no conscience' actually means 'weak or dysfunctional' conscience." Therefore, a truth-seeker must appeal to the conscience, meaning, "make the conscience work out, make it work right, and make it do all the work." True Confessions is a manual for anyone whose job it is to get the truth. For example, Human Resources personnel during the job interview process or Law Enforcement interviewers who can use Arcaro's theories to open a window into the psyche of a suspect under interrogation.

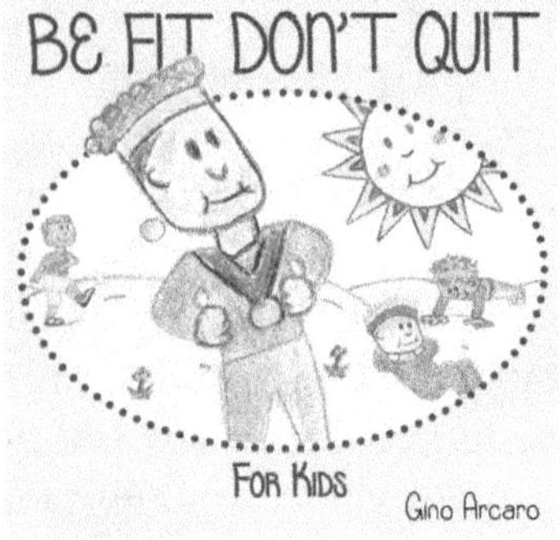

Be Fit Don't Quit

Full of exercise ideas young children can try on their own or with a parent, this book will rekindle in any adult a love for the simple act of playing. Gino Arcaro has spent his life working out and teaching young adults about the importance of "being fit." He wrote Be Fit Don't Quit to express a tried-and-true message: Exercising is natural and fun. Never quit!

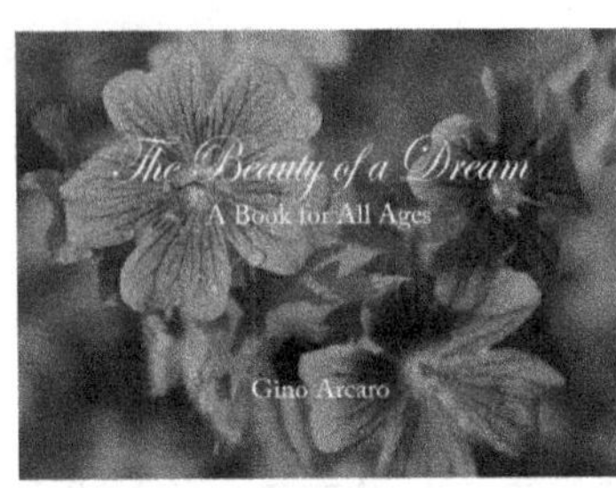

Beauty of a Dream

Inspired by the birth of his first grandchild, Arcaro wrote this colour picture-infused booklet to encourage the reader to dream, dream big and never stop dreaming. "No one can break into your dream and rob you of it, unless you let them." His message, in this book as in all his works, is a challenge for the reader to strive to reach his/her potential and make an impact in this world. A perfect gift for someone in your life who needs to be "lifted" or reminded that dreaming is important!

www.ingramcontent.com/pod-product-compliance
Lightning Source LLC
Chambersburg PA
CBHW081654270326
41933CB00017B/3165